SOAP
for
Emergency Medicine

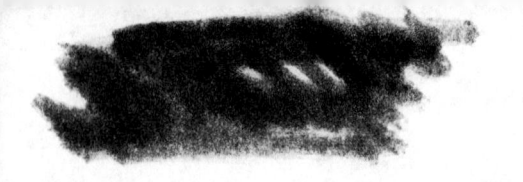

Look for other books in this series!

SOAP for Obstetrics and Gynecology

SOAP for Pediatrics

SOAP for Family Medicine

SOAP for Internal Medicine

SOAP for Urology

SOAP for Dermatology

SOAP for Neurology

SOAP
for
Emergency Medicine

Michael C. Bond, MD
Resident, Emergency Medicine/Internal Medicine
Allegheny General Hospital
Pittsburgh, Pennsylvania

Series Editor:
Peter S. Uzelac, MD, FACOG
Assistant Professor
Department of Obstetrics and Gynecology
University of Southern California Keck School of Medicine
Los Angeles, California

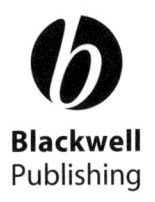

Blackwell
Publishing

© 2005 Blackwell Publishing, Inc.

Blackwell Publishing, Inc., 350 Main Street, Malden, Massachusetts 02148-5018, USA
Blackwell Publishing Ltd, 9600 Garsington Road, Oxford OX4 2DQ, UK
Blackwell Publishing Asia Pty Ltd, 550 Swanston Street, Carlton, Victoria 3053, Australia

All rights reserved. No part of this publication may be reproduced in any form or by any electronic or mechanical means, including information storage and retrieval systems, without permission in writing from the publisher, except by a reviewer who may quote brief passages in a review.

04 05 06 07 5 4 3 2 1

ISBN: 1-4051-0442-2

Library of Congress Cataloging-in-Publication Data

Bond, Michael C.
    SOAP for emergency medicine / Michael C. Bond.
      p. ; cm.
    Includes index.
    ISBN 1-4051-0442-2 (pbk.)
    1. Emergency medicine—Handbooks, manuals, etc.
    [DNLM: 1. Emergency Medicine—Handbooks. WB 39 B711s 2005]   I. Title.
    RC86.8.B66   2005
    616.02′5—dc22

                                                2004006158

A catalogue record for this title is available from the British Library

Acquisitions: Beverly Copland
Development: Selene Steneck
Production: Jennifer Kowalewski
Cover and Interior design: Meral Dabrovich
Typesetter: TechBooks in New Delhi, India
Printed and bound by Sheridan Books in Ann Arbor, MI

For further information on Blackwell Publishing, visit our website:
  www.blackwellmedstudent.com

Notice: The indications and dosages of all drugs in this book have been recommended in the medical literature and conform to the practices of the general community. The medications described do not necessarily have specific approval by the Food and Drug Administration for use in the diseases and dosages for which they are recommended. The package insert for each drug should be consulted for use and dosage as approved by the FDA. Because standards for usage change, it is advisable to keep abreast of revised recommendations, particularly those concerning new drugs.

The publisher's policy is to use permanent paper from mills that operate a sustainable forestry policy, and which has been manufactured from pulp processed using acid-free and elementary chlorine-free practices. Furthermore, the publisher ensures that the text paper and cover board used have met acceptable environmental accreditation standards.

This book is dedicated to my wife, Ginger, for all that she has done, and continues to do to support me in my academic and professional pursuits. I love you.

Contents

To the Reader	xi
Acknowledgments	xii
Consultant	xiii
Reviewers	xiv
Abbreviations	xv
Normal Lab Values	xix

I. Cardiology — 1
1. Aortic Dissection — 2
2. Bradycardia/Complete Heart Block — 4
3. Cardiac Arrest — 6
4. Chest Pain — 8
5. Congestive Heart Failure — 10
6. Endocarditis — 12
7. Hypertensive Crisis — 14
8. Myocardial Infarction — 16
9. Palpitations — 18
10. Syncope — 20
11. Unstable Angina — 22
12. Venous Thrombosis — 24

II. Hematology — 27
13. Anemia — 28
14. ITP/TTP — 30
15. Sickle Cell Disease — 32

III. Endocrine — 35
16. Diabetic Ketoacidosis — 36
17. Hypoglycemia — 38

IV. Pulmonary — 41
18. Asthma Exacerbation — 42
19. COPD Exacerbation — 44
20. Pleural Effusion — 46
21. Pneumonia — 48
22. Pneumothorax — 50
23. Pulmonary Edema — 52
24. Pulmonary Embolism — 54

V. Gastrointestinal — 57
25. Abdominal Aortic Aneurysm — 58
26. Appendicitis — 60
27. Bowel Obstruction — 62
28. Biliary Disease — 64
29. Diarrhea — 66
30. Diverticulitis — 68

31. Foreign-Body Ingestion — 70
32. Gastroesophageal Reflux Disease — 72
33. Gastrointestinal Bleeding — 74
34. Hepatitis — 76
35. Ischemic Bowel — 78
36. Pancreatitis — 80
37. Peptic Ulcer Disease — 82

VI. HEENT — 85
38. Conjunctivitis — 86
39. Corneal Abrasion — 88
40. Dysphagia — 90
41. Epistaxis — 92
42. Otitis Externa — 94
43. Otitis Media — 96
44. Pharyngitis — 98
45. Toothache/Fractured Tooth — 100

VII. Genitourinary — 103
46. Acute Renal Failure — 104
47. Epididymitis — 106
48. Hernia — 108
49. Hydrocele/Varicocele — 110
50. Kidney Stones/Nephrolithiasis — 112
51. Pyelonephritis/UTI — 114
52. Rhabdomyolysis — 116
53. STD — 118
54. Testicular Torsion — 120

VIII. OB/GYN — 123
55. Ectopic Pregnancy — 124
56. Ovarian Torsion/Cyst — 126
57. Pregnancy — 128
58. Pelvic Inflammatory Disease — 130
59. Sexual Assault — 132
60. Spontaneous Abortion ("Miscarriage") — 134
61. Vaginal Bleeding — 136
62. Vulvovaginitis — 138

IX. Neurology — 141
63. Altered Mental Status — 142
64. Headache — 144
65. Meningitis — 146
66. Seizures — 148
67. Stroke — 150
68. Vertigo — 152
69. Weakness — 154

X. Trauma   157
- 70. Animal Bite   158
- 71. Ankle Sprain   160
- 72. Burns   162
- 73. Fracture   164
- 74. Head Injury   166
- 75. Laceration   168
- 76. Low Back Pain   170
- 77. Wrist Pain   172

XI. Psychiatry   175
- 78. Overdose   176
- 79. Psychiatric Evaluation   178

XII. Dermatology   181
- 80. Contact Dermatitis   182
- 81. Urticaria   184

XIII. Pediatrics   187
- 82. Abdominal Pain   188
- 83. Febrile Seizures   190
- 84. Fever of Unknown Origin   192
- 85. Gastroenteritis   194

Index   **197**

To the Reader

Like most medical students, I started my ward experience head down and running, eager to finally make contact with real patients. What I found was a confusing world, completely different from anything I had known during the first two years of medical school. New language, foreign abbreviations, and residents too busy to set my bearings straight: Where would I begin?

Pocket textbooks, offering medical knowledge in a convenient and portable package, seemed to be the logical solution. Unfortunately, I found myself spending valuable time sifting through large amounts of text, often not finding the answer to my question, and in the process, missing out on teaching points during rounds!

I designed the SOAP series to provide medical students and house staff with pocket manuals that truly serve their intended purpose: quick accessibility to the most practical clinical information in a user-friendly format. At the inception of this project, I envisioned all of the benefits the SOAP format would bring to the reader:

- Learning through this model reinforces a thought process that is already familiar to students and residents, facilitating easier long-term retention.

- SOAP promotes good communication between physicians and facilitates the teaching/learning process.

- SOAP puts the emphasis back on the patient's clinical problem and not the diagnosis.

- In the age of managed care, SOAP meets the challenge of providing efficiency while maintaining quality.

- As sound medical-legal practice gains attention in physician training, SOAP emphasizes adherence to a documentation style that leaves little room for potential misinterpretation.

Rather than attempting to summarize the contents of a thousand-page textbook into a miniature form, the SOAP series focuses exclusively on guidance through patient encounters. In a typical use, "finding out where to start" or "refreshing your memory" with SOAP books should be possible in less than a minute. Subjects are always confined to two pages, and the most important points have been highlighted. Topics have been limited to those problems you will most commonly encounter repeatedly during your training, and contents are grouped according to the hospital or clinic setting. Facts and figures that are not particularly helpful to surviving life on the wards, such as demographics, pathophysiology, and busy tables and graphs have purposely been omitted (such details are much better studied in a quiet environment using large and comprehensive texts).

Congratulations on your achievements thus far, and I wish you a highly successful medical career!

Peter S. Uzelac, MD, FACOG

Acknowledgments

I must thank the staff at Blackwell Publishing, especially Bev Copland and Selene Steneck, who were instrumental in walking me through the entire process of creating this book.

I would like to thank the residency program at Allegheny General Hospital for providing an environment rich in teaching, providing me with the knowledge from which this book is written, and being supportive throughout the entire process.

Last, but certainly not least, I want to acknowledge the continued undying support and guidance from my wife, Ginger.

Consultant

Nick E. Colovos, MD, FAAEM
Director of Emergency Medical Services
Department of Emergency Medicine
Allegheny General Hospital
Pittsburgh, Pennsylvania
Assistant Professor of Emergency Medicine
Drexel University College of Medicine
Philadelphia, Pennsylvania

Reviewers

Brenda Grant
Class of 2005
Texas Tech University Health Sciences Center School of Medicine
El Paso, Texas

Andrew Louie
Class of 2004
George Washington University School of Medicine
Washington, DC

Billy K. Parsley
Class of 2004
University of Tennessee Health Science Center College of Medicine
Memphis, Tennessee

Mai B. Tran
Class of 2004
Western University of Health Sciences
Pomona, California

Kavid Nik Udompanyanan
Class of 2004
Harvard University School of Medicine
Boston, Massachusetts

Abbreviations

AAA	abdominal aortic aneurysm
ABG	arterial blood gas
ACE	angiotensin-converting enzyme
ACLS	advanced cardiac life support
ALS	amyotrophic lateral sclerosis (Lou Gehrig's disease)
ALT	alanine aminotransferase
ARDS	adult respiratory distress syndrome
ASAP	as soon as possible
AST	aspartate aminotransferase
ATFL	anterior talofibular ligament
ATN	acute tubular necosis
AV	atrioventricular
β-hCG	beta human chorionic gonadotropin
bid	*bis in die* (twice daily)
BNP	B-type natriuretic peptide
bpm	beats per minute
BUN	blood urea nitrogen
Ca	calcium
CABG	coronary artery bypass graft
CAD	coronary atherosclerotic disease
CAP	community-acquired pneumonia
CBC	complete blood count
CHF	congestive heart failure
CK	creatinine kinase
CKMB	creatinine kinase MB
CMT	cervical motion tenderness
CNS	central nervous system
COPD	chronic obstructive pulmonary disease
COX-2	cyclooxygenase 2
CPAP	continuous positive airway pressure
CPR	cardiopulmonary resuscitation
CRP	C-reactive protein
CSF	cerebrospinal fluid
CT	computed tomography
CTS	carpal tunnel syndrome
CXR	chest x-ray
CVA	cerebrovascular accident; costovertebral angle
DIC	disseminated intravascular coagulation
DKA	diabetic ketoacidosis
D50	50% dextrose solution
DVT	deep venous thrombosis
DUB	dysfunctional uterine bleeding
ECG	electrocardiogram
ED	emergency department
EDH	epidural hematoma
EEG	electroencephalogram
ELISA	enzyme-linked immunosorbent assay

ELS	Eaton-Lambert syndrome
ENT	ears, nose, throat
EP	electrophysiology
ESR	erythrocyte sedimentation rate
EtOH	ethanol
GERD	gastroesophageal reflux disease
GI	gastrointestinal
Gluc	glucose
GU	genitourinary
Gyn	gynecology
HAV	hepatitis A virus
Hb	hemoglobin
HBV	hepatitis B virus
HCT	hematocrit
HCV	hepatitis C virus
HCG	human chorionic gonadotropin
HEENT	head, ears, eyes, nose, throat
HELLP	hemolysis, elevated liver enzymes, low platelets
HIB	*Haemophilus influenzae* B
HIDA	hepatobiliary iminodiacetic acid
HIV	human immunodeficiency virus
hr	hour
HSV	herpes simplex virus
HTN	hypertension
ICB	intracranial bleed
ICU	intensive care unit
IgG	immunoglobulin G
IgM	immunoglobulin M
IM	intramuscular
IMA	inferior mesenteric artery
INR	international normalized ratio
IS	infantile spasm
ITP	idiopathic thrombocytopenic purpura
IUP	intrauterine pregnancy
IV	intravenous
IVC	inferior vena cava
IVDA	intravenous drug abuse
IVF	intravenous fluid
IVIG	intravenous immunoglobulin
IVP	intravenous pyelogram
KOH	potassium hydroxide
LDH	lactate dehydrogenase
LES	lower esophageal sphincter
LFT	liver function test
LMWH	low-molecular-weight heparin
LOC	loss of consciousness
MDI	metered-dose inhaler
MG	myasthenia gravis
MI	myocardial infarction
MNF	monitored nursing floor

MRI	magnetic resonance imaging
MS	multiple sclerosis
Na	sodium
NG	nasogastric
NICU	neonatal intensive care unit
NKH	nonketotic hyperglycemia
NPO	*nulla per os* (nothing by mouth)
NQWMI	non-Q-wave myocardial infarction
NSAID	nonsteroidal anti-inflammatory drug
NSS	normal saline solution
Ob/Gyn	Obstetrics/Gynecology
OKT3	anti-CD3 monoclonal antibody
OMFS	oral and maxillofacial surgery
OR	operating room
OTC	over-the-counter
PaO$_2$	arterial partial pressure of oxygen
PE	pulmonary embolism
PCP	primary care provider
PID	pelvic inflammatory disease
PO	*per os* (by mouth)
PRBCs	packed red blood cells
PMH	past medical history
PQRST	place, quality, radiation, symptoms, timing
pt	patient
PT	prothrombin time
PTCA	percutaneous coronary angioplasty
PTT	partial thromboplastin time
PUD	peptic ulcer disease
qd	*quaque die* (once daily)
qhs	*quaque hora somni* (every night)
RBC	red blood cell
RICE	rest, ice, compression, and elevation
RLQ	right lower quadrant of abdomen
RPR	rapid plasma reagin
RUQ	right upper quadrant of abdomen
RV	right ventricle
SA	sinoatrial
SAH	subarachnoid hemorrhage
SBP	systolic blood pressure
SCD	sickle cell disease
SDH	subdural hematoma
SLR	straight leg raise
SpO$_2$	oxygen saturation by pulse oximeter
SSRI	selective serotonin reuptake inhibitor
STD	sexually transmitted disease
TCAs	tricyclic antidepressants
TEE	transesophageal echocardiogram
TIA	transient ischemic attack
TIBC	total iron-binding capacity
TM	tympanic membrane

TMP-SMX	trimethoprim-sulfamethoxazole
TOA	tubo-ovarian abscess
Trop-I	troponin I
TSH	thyroid-stimulating hormone
TTE	transthoracic echocardiogram
TTP	thrombotic thrombocytopenic purpura
UA	urinalysis
UTI	urinary tract infection
UV	ultraviolet
VTach	ventricular tachycardia
WBC	white blood cell
WHO	World Health Organization
wk	week

Normal Lab Values

Blood, Plasma, Serum

Aminotransferase, alanine (ALT, SGPT)	0–35 U/L
Aminotransferase, aspartate (AST, SGOT)	0–35 U/L
Ammonia, plasma	40–80 μg/dL
Amylase, serum	0–130 U/L
Antistreptolysin O titer	Less than 150 units
Bicarbonate, serum	23–28 meq/L
Bilirubin, serum	
Total	0.3–1.2 mg/dL
Direct	0–0.3 mg/dL
Blood gases, arterial (room air)	
P_{O_2}	80–100 mm Hg
P_{CO_2}	35–45 mm Hg
pH	7.38–7.44
Calcium, serum	9–10.5 mg/dL
Carbon dioxide content, serum	23–28 meq/L
Chloride, serum	98–106 meq/L
Cholesterol, total, plasma	150–199 mg/dL (desirable)
Cholesterol, low-density lipoprotein (LDL), plasma	$\leq$ 130 mg/dL (desirable)
Cholesterol, high-density lipoprotein (HDL), plasma	$\geq$ 40 mg/dL (desirable)
Complement, serum	
C3	55–120 mg/dL
Total	37–55 U/mL
Copper, serum	70–155 μg/dL
Creatine kinase, serum	30–170 U/L
Creatinine, serum	0.7–1.3 mg/dL
Ethanol, blood	< 50 mg/dL
Fibrinogen, plasma	150–350 mg/dL
Folate, red cell	160–855 ng/mL
Folate, serum	2.5–20 ng/mL
Glucose, plasma	
Fasting	70–105 mg/dL
2 hours postprandial	< 140 mg/dL
Iron, serum	0–160 μg/dL
Iron binding capacity, serum	250–460 μg/dL
Lactate dehydrogenase, serum	60–100 U/L
Lactic acid, venous blood	6–16 mg/dL
Lead, blood	< 40 μg/dL

Lipase, serum	< 95 U/L
Magnesium, serum	1.5–2.4 mg/dL
Manganese, serum	0.3–0.9 ng/mL
Methylmalonic acid, serum	150–370 nmol/L
Osmolality plasma	275–295 mosm/kg H_2O
Phosphatase, acid, serum	0.5–5.5 U/L
Phosphatase, alkaline, serum	36–92 U/L
Phosphorus, inorganic, serum	3–4.5 mg/dL
Potassium, serum	3.5–5 meq/L
Protein, serum	
Total	6.0–7.8 g/dL
Albumin	3.5–5.5 g/dL
Globulins	2.5–3.5 g/dL
Alpha$_1$	0.2–0.4 g/dL
Alpha$_2$	0.5–0.9 g/dL
Beta	0.6–1.1 g/dL
Gamma	0.7–1.7 g/dL
Rheumatoid factor	< 40 U/mL
Sodium, serum	136–145 meq/L
Triglycerides	< 250 mg/dL (desirable)
Urea nitrogen, serum	8–20 mg/dL
Uric acid, serum	2.5–8 mg/dL
Vitamin B_{12}, serum	200–800 pg/mL

Cerebrospinal Fluid

Cell count	0–5 cells/μL
Glucose (less than 40% of simultaneous plasma concentration is abnormal)	40–80 mg/dL
Protein	15–60 mg/dL
Pressure (opening)	70–200 mm H_2O

Endocrine

Adrenocorticotropin (ACTH)	9–52 pg/mL
Aldosterone, serum	
Supine	2–5 ng/dL
Standing	7–20 ng/dL
Aldosterone, urine	5–19 μg/24 h
Cortisol	
Serum 8 AM	8–20 μg/dL
5 PM	3–13 μg/dL

1 h after cosyntropin usually ≥ 8 μg/dL above baseline	> 18 μg/dL
overnight suppression test	< 5 μg/dL
Urine free cortisol	< 90 μg/24 h
Estradiol, serum	
Male	10–30 pg/mL
Female	
Cycle day 1–10	50–100 pmol/L
Cycle day 11–20	50–200 pmol/L
Cycle day 21–30	70–150 pmol/L
Estriol, urine	> 12 mg/24 h
Follicle-stimulating hormone, serum	
Male (adult)	5–15 mU/mL
Female	
Follicular or luteal phase	5–20 mU/mL
Midcycle peak	30–50 mU/mL
Postmenopausal	> 35 mU/mL
Insulin, serum (fasting)	5–20 mU/L
17-ketosteroids, urine	
Male	8–22 mg/24 h
Female	Up to 15 μg/24 h
Luteinizing hormone, serum	
Male	3–15 mU/mL (3–15 U/L)
Female	
Follicular or luteal phase	5–22 mU/mL
Midcycle peak	30–250 mU/mL
Postmenopausal	> 30 mU/mL
Parathyroid hormone, serum	10–65 pg/mL
Progesterone	
Luteal	3–30 ng/mL
Follicular	< 1 ng/mL
Prolactin, serum	
Male	< 15 ng/mL
Female	< 20 ng/mL
Testosterone, serum	
Adult male	300–1200 ng/dL
Female	20–75 ng/dL
Thyroid function tests (normal ranges vary)	
Thyroid iodine (^{131}I) uptake	10% to 30% of administered dose at 24 h

Thyroid-stimulating hormone (TSH)	0.5–5.0 μU/mL
Thyroxine (T4), serum	
Total	5–12 pg/dL
Free	0.9–2.4 ng/dL
Free T4 index	4–11
Triiodothyronine, resin (T3)	25%–35%
Triiodothyronine, serum (T3)	70–195 ng/dL
Vitamin D	
1,25-dihydroxy, serum	25–65 pg/mL
25-hydroxy, serum	15–80 ng/mL

Gastrointestinal

Fecal urobilinogen	40–280 mg/24 h
Gastrin, serum	0–180 pg/mL
Lactose tolerance test	
Increase in plasma glucose	> 15 mg/dL
Lipase, ascitic fluid	< 200 U/L
Secretin-cholecystokinin pancreatic function	> 80 meq/L of HCO_3 in at least 1 specimen collected over 1 h
Stool fat	< 5 g/d on a 100-g fat diet
Stool nitrogen	< 2 g/d
Stool weight	< 200 g/d

Hematology

Activated partial thromboplastin time	25–35 s
Bleeding time	< 10 min
Coagulation factors, plasma	
Factor I	150–350 mg/dL
Factor II	60%–150% of normal
Factor V	60%–150% of normal
Factor VII	60%–150% of normal
Factor VIII	60%–150% of normal
Factor IX	60%–150% of normal
Factor X	60%–150% of normal
Factor XI	60%–150% of normal
Factor XII	60%–150% of normal
Erythrocyte count	4.2–5.9 million cells/μL
Erythropoietin	< 30 mU/mL
D-dimer	< 0.5 μg/mL
Ferritin, serum	15–200 ng/mL

Glucose-6-phosphate dehydrogenase, blood	5–15 U/g Hgb
Haptoglobin, serum	50–150 mg/dL
Hematocrit	
Male	41%–51%
Female	36%–47%
Hemoglobin, blood	
Male	14–17 g/dL
Female	12–16 g/dL
Hemoglobin, plasma	0.5–5 mg/dL
Leukocyte alkaline phosphatase	15–40 mg of phosphorus liberated/h per 10^{10} cells
Score	13–130/100 polymorphonuclear neutrophils and band forms
Leukocyte count	
Nonblacks	4000–10,000/μL
Blacks	3500–10,000/μL
Lymphocytes	
CD4+ cell count	640–1175/μL
CD8+ cell count	335–875/μL
CD4 : CD8 ratio	1.0–4.0
Mean corpuscular hemoglobin (MCH)	28–32 pg
Mean corpuscular hemoglobin concentration (MCHC)	32–36 g/dL
Mean corpuscular volume (MCV)	80–100 fL
Platelet count	150,000–350,000/μL
Protein C activity, plasma	67%–131%
Protein C resistance	2.2–2.6
Protein S activity, plasma	82%–144%
Prothrombin time	11–13 s
Reticulocyte count	0.5%–1.5% of erythrocytes
Absolute	23,000–90,000 cells/μL
Schilling test (oral administration of radioactive cobalamin-labeled vitamin B_{12})	8.5%–28% excreted in urine per 24–48 h
Sedimentation rate, erythrocyte (Westergren)	
Male	0–15 mm/h
Female	0–20 mm/h

Volume, blood
  Plasma
    Male   25–44 mL/kg body weight
    Female   28–43 mL/kg body weight
  Erythrocyte
    Male   25–35 mL/kg body weight
    Female   20–30 mL/kg body weight

Urine

Amino acids	200–400 mg/24 h
Amylase	6.5–48.1 U/h
Calcium	100–300 mg/d on unrestricted diet
Chloride	80–250 meq/d (varies with intake)
Copper	0–100 μg/24 h
Creatine	
Male	4–40 mg/24 h
Female	0–100 mg/24 h
Creatinine	15–25 mg/kg per 24 h
Creatinine clearance	90–140 mL/min
Osmolality	38–1400 mosm/kg H_2O
Phosphate, tubular resorption	79%–94% (0.79–0.94) of filtered load
Potassium	25–100 meq/24 h (varies with intake)
Protein	< 100 mg/24 h
Sodium	100–260 meq/24h (varies with intake)
Uric acid	250–750 mg/24 h (varies with diet)
Urobilinogen	0.05–2.5 mg/24 h

I
Cardiology

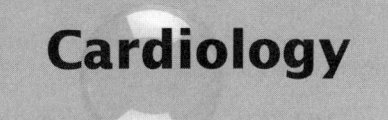

Aortic Dissection

S **Determine the onset of the pt's symptoms**
What are the pt's current symptoms?
Pts typically complain of acute onset of tearing chest pain that radiates to the back.
Approximately 10% of cases may be asymptomatic.
Other symptoms include hoarseness, syncope, nausea/vomiting, abdominal pain, and paralysis.

Does the pt have any neurologic symptoms?
Weakness, numbness, or cerebrovascular accident (CVA) symptoms may represent an extension of the dissection into the carotid arteries.
Pts with CVA symptoms are more likely to have painless dissection, which may be a result of their inability to report their pain.

Does the pt have any risk factors for aortic dissection?
- Hypertension (most common)
- Pregnancy
- Atherosclerosis
- Aortic coarctation
- Marfan's syndrome
- Smoking
- Connective tissue disorders
- Diabetes
- Tertiary syphilis
- Cocaine abuse
- Recent cardiac catheterization or cardiac surgery
- Males are 10 times more likely to suffer a dissection.

Obtain a past medical history
Obtain a list of the pt's current medications
Have they changed, missed, or stopped any of their current medications? This may result in rebound hypertension leading to the dissection.
Is the pt taking any herbal supplements? Several herbs (e.g., ephedra) can cause hypertension (HTN).

Perform a general review of symptoms
May suggest diagnosis of esophageal spasm, gastroesophageal reflux disease, peptic ulcer disease, or pericarditis.

O **Check vital signs**
Elevated blood pressure and/or heart rate can exacerbate the dissection.

Perform a physical exam
Cardiac: Note aortic heart sounds. Is there a diastolic murmur of aortic insufficiency? Pericardial rub?
- A new murmur may signify that the dissection has compromised the heart valve.
Carotid: Listen for bruits, which may indicate turbulent flow caused by vessel wall abnormalities.
Neurologic: Check for focal deficits and mental status changes.

Obtain an ECG
Used to exclude myocardial infarction from the diagnosis, although the dissection can extend into the coronary arteries, causing ischemia.
Signs of left ventricular hypertrophy may support the diagnosis of long-term HTN.

Obtain a CXR
CXR is 90% sensitive for aortic dissection. May see a widened mediastinum, blurred aortic knob, an aortic double density, deviation of trachea, or pleural effusion.

Obtain a diagnostic study

Chest CT scan, MRI, and TEE all approach 100% in sensitivity and specificity for dissection.

Choice of exam depends on availability and expertise at your individual hospital.
- MRI, when available, is less invasive. However, it may be difficult to obtain in the critically ill pt.
- TEE, although invasive, is ideal for the critically ill pt because it can be done at bedside.
- Chest CT requires IV contrast and will require premedication if pt has an iodine allergy.
- If suspicion is high, two negative diagnostic studies are needed to exclude the diagnosis.

A ### Aortic Dissection
Aortic dissection is a tear in the aortic intima, where blood passes into the aortic media, thereby separating the intima from the surrounding media and/or adventitia, and creating a false lumen.

Differential Diagnosis
- Myocardial infarction
- Acute pericarditis
- Peptic ulcer disease
- Pulmonary embolus
- Pneumothorax
- Esophageal spasm

P ### Immediate blood pressure lowering and control of heart rate is needed

An elevated blood pressure and tachycardia increase the shear forces on the aorta.
A goal of a systolic blood pressure less than 120 mm Hg should be achieved.
Initial therapy consists of β-blockers or Ca channel blockers.
Add vasodilators (e.g., nitroprusside) if blood pressure remains elevated.
- Monitor heart rate closely because reflex tachycardia may result from the use of vasodilators.

Provide pain relief
Narcotics are preferred.

Diagnostic study will dictate whether operative intervention is needed
Stanford Type A
- All dissections involving the proximal (ascending) aorta
- 70% of aortic dissections
- Has a greater risk for complication with extension into carotid/coronary arteries.
- Requires surgical repair. Consult cardiothoracic surgeon.
- Mortality rate increases 1% per hour during the first 48 hours.
- Worse prognosis than Type B

Stanford Type B
- Dissection involving the distal (descending) aorta only
- 30% of dissections
- Greater likelihood of being successfully managed medically.
- Surgical repair needed if there is evidence of extension into the renal or mesenteric arteries as seen by renal failure and/or mesenteric ischemia.

Admit pt to the ICU

Bradycardia/Complete Heart Block — Cardiology

S   Determine whether the pt has any symptoms
Some pts have no symptoms and are only found to have complete heart block or bradycardia on a routine physical exam or ECG.
Pts may complain of lightheadedness, palpitations, dyspnea, chest pain, syncope, or mental status changes.

Has the pt been started on any new medications or were any doses increased?
β-blockers, Ca channel blockers, tricyclic antidepressants (TCAs), and digoxin may all cause atrioventricular (AV) node block and lead to bradycardia.
Amiodarone and clonidine toxicity can present with bradycardia.
Determine whether the pt may have inadvertently taken too much medication.

Does the pt have a history of coronary atherosclerotic disease (CAD) or myocardial infarction (MI)?
Progression of CAD and MI can cause complete heart block.

Has the pt fallen, had a recent stroke, or suffered a head injury?
Increased intracranial pressure due to intracerebral hemorrhage, cerebrovascular accident, or subarachnoid hemorrhage can cause heart block.

Does the pt have any history of amyloidosis or sarcoidosis?
This disease can infiltrate the sinoatrial (SA) and AV nodes, leading to heart block.

Has the pt traveled or been outdoors recently?
Chagas' disease and Lyme disease cause heart block.

Perform a general review of symptoms
This may help elicit any potential medical problems complicating the heart block.
Weight gain and/or cold intolerance may suggest hypothyroidism, a potentially reversible cause of heart block.

O   Perform a physical exam
Thyroid: Check for masses or thyroidomegaly.
Neck: Measure jugular venous distention. Cannon A waves can be seen in complete heart block.
Cardiac: Listen for murmurs, irregular pulse, S3 or S4 as signs of congestive heart failure.
Lungs: Listen for crackles, a sign of heart failure.
Neurologic: Check for focal deficits or mental status changes.

Check orthostatics
Evaluate whether the pt is able to compensate with a faster heart rate.
Use caution if pt complains of lightheadedness or has had a syncopal episode.

Check the ECG
Pay particular attention to the P waves and PR interval.
- 1st-degree heart block: PR interval constant but > 0.2 sec.
- 2nd-degree heart block:
  - (Mobitz I – Wenkebach): Progressively prolonged PR interval with an intermittent nonconducted P wave.
  - (Mobitz II): constant PR interval with intermittent non-conducted P waves.
- 3rd-degree heart block: P waves are not conducted and not related to the QRS complex.

Attempt to differentiate whether the pt has sinus bradycardia, 1st-, 2nd-, or 3rd-degree heart block.
Evaluate for left bundle branch or right bundle branch blocks.

Check the following labs
Cardiac enzymes to rule out recent cardiac ischemia or myocardial infarction.
TSH to rule out hypothyroidism.
Digoxin level and/or urine drug screen to check for TCA use.

A

Sinus bradycardia
Heart rate < 60 bpm

1st-degree heart block
A PR duration [time from the end of the P wave to the beginning of the QRS complex] > 200 milliseconds (1 large box on ECG paper)

2nd-degree heart block
An atrioventricular block where an occasional impulse from the atria does not propragate to the ventricules, resulting in a missed beat

3rd-degree heart block (complete heart block)
Complete electrical dissociation between the atrium and the ventricles

P

If pt is asymptomatic, observation and discontinuation of any agents that may block the AV node (e.g., β-blockers, Ca channel blockers, digoxin, TCAs) is all that is needed

If pt is symptomatic, consider the following
Administer atropine.
- Increases SA and AV nodal conduction.
- Not effective if pt has had a heart transplant.

Administer epinephrine.
- Used if pt is in asystole or has continued symptomatic bradycardia despite atropine use.

Place transcutaneous pacemaker leads on pt and start pacing if medical management fails.
Place transvenous pacemaker if above measures fail.

If bradycardia is caused by a medication overdose and pt is symptomatic, administer

IM or IV glucagon for β-blocker overdose
IV Ca for Ca channel blocker overdose
Digoxin-specific antibody fragments for digoxin overdose (typically restricted to life-threatening toxicity only)

Arrange admission to a monitored nursing floor or coronary care unit

Cardiac Arrest — Cardiology

S **Determine how long the pt has been in cardiac arrest**
Determine how long the pt was unconscious before CPR was initiated
A delay of more than 5 minutes is generally associated with major neurologic injury.
Witnessed arrest and immediate initiation of CPR improves outcomes.

Obtain a quick past medical history
Does the pt have a history of sudden cardiac death or arrhythmias?
- Recurrent arrhythmia

Has the pt had a myocardial infarction (MI) in the past or a coronary artery bypass graft or percutaneous coronary angioplasty (PTCA)?
- Possible acute myocardial infarction

Does the pt have a history of depression or suicide attempts?
- Hints at a possible overdose and repeat suicide attempt

Does the pt have a known code status?
What was the pt doing before arresting?
If eating, pt may have choked and had a primary respiratory arrest.
If pt was working on his house or car, he might have been electrocuted.

Did the pt complain of any pain or other symptoms before arresting?
Lightheadedness, palpitations, or a racing heartbeat suggest an arrhythmia as cause.
Chest pain may be seen with MI or pulmonary embolism (PE).
Shortness of breath is also associated with MI and PE.

Is the pt a victim of a recent trauma?
Internal injuries and exsanguination need to be ruled out.

Does the pt have any risk factor for PE?
See Pulmonary Embolism, p. 54

O **Ventilate the pt with a bag-valve-mask or intubate**
Quickly place pt on a monitor and determine the underlying rhythm
Pts in ventricular fibrillation or ventricular tachycardia have the greatest survival rate if they are defibrillated early.
Follow the appropriate advanced cardiac life support (ACLS) algorithm.
If pt has a normal rhythm on the monitor, think of potential treatable causes for pulseless electrical activity:

- Hypovolemia	- Acidosis	- Cardiac tamponade
- Hypo-/Hyperkalemia	- Hypothermia	- Pulmonary embolism
- Hypoxemia	- Overdose	- Tension pneumothorax

Initiate chest compressions and check frequently for a spontaneous pulse
Perform a physical exam
Look closely for signs of trauma or drug use.
Ensure that the pt has equal breath sounds bilaterally.
Note any tracheal deviation as a sign of tension pneumothorax.

If concerned about hypothermia, check a core body temperature
Establish venous access to administer medications
If unable to obtain venous access, the following medications can be administered down the endotracheal tube:

- Epinephrine
- Lidocaine
- Atropine
- Narcan

Obtain a CXR
Look for signs of pneumothorax, enlarged cardiac silhouette as a surrogate marker for cardiac tamponade, and any rib fractures.

Obtain an ECG
If signs of an acute MI are present, pt needs to be taken to cardiac catherization lab ASAP. Thrombolytics are contraindicated with prolonged chest compressions.

Check the following labs
Cardiac enzymes to rule out ischemia.
Full set of electrolytes to exclude any major electrolyte disturbance.
CBC to exclude anemia.
ABG to demonstrate whether the pt has been oxygenated well and if he has a normal pH.

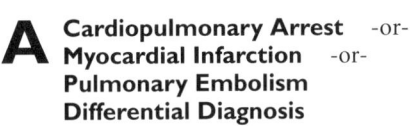

A
Cardiopulmonary Arrest -or-
Myocardial Infarction -or-
Pulmonary Embolism
Differential Diagnosis
     - Overdose   - Cerebrovascular accident

P
Follow ACLS protocols
Treat underlying disorders
Replace electrolytes immediately.
If pt has hyperkalemia, immediately administer (all of the following):
- Ca gluconate   - D50
- IV insulin   - Kayexalate

If overdose, treat accordingly.
If hypovolemic or hemorrhaging, treat aggressively with IV hydration and/or administer packed red blood cells.

If pt is having a myocardial infarction
If possible, make arrangements for immediate PTCA.
Thrombolytics are typically contraindicated because of the risk of bleeding post-CPR.

If unable to establish a perfusable rhythm within 30 to 60 minutes, the pt is typically pronounced dead
Follow local guidelines concerning the notification of your local coroner or medical examiner.

Arrange for admission to the coronary care unit
If normal circulation is restored.

S — Determine the PQRST of the pain

P = Place of the pain. Determine its exact location.
Q = Quality of the pain. Rate it on a scale of 1 to 10 (10 being the worst), and ask the pt to describe it (e.g., sharp, dull, pressure, burning).
R = Radiation. Does the pain radiate to the jaw, shoulder, stomach, or back?
- Pain radiating to jaw or left shoulder is common with cardiac ischemia.
- Pain radiating to back should increase suspicion for aortic dissection.

S = associated Symptoms. What makes the pain worse or better (e.g., bending over, walking up stairs, lying down, resting, eating, etc.)?
T = Timing. How long has the pain been present, or how long does it last when it occurs?
- Fleeting pain that lasts seconds is typically musculoskeletal in origin.

Does the pt have any risk factors for myocardial infarction?
See Myocardial Infarction p. 16

Has the pt experienced any symptoms consistent with angina?
Exertional shortness of breath or chest pain

Has there been any trauma, heavy lifting, or heavy exertion?
More consistent with musculoskeletal chest wall pain

Determine the presence of cough, fever, or upper respiratory symptoms
More consistent with pneumonia, pleurisy, or costochondritis

Does the pt have a history of gastroesophageal reflux disease (GERD) or esophageal spasm?
Esophageal irritation from GERD or spasm can present as severe chest pain. Typically, pain is either exacerbated or relieved by eating.

Does the pt have a history of chronic obstructive pulmonary disease/asthma?
Chest pain can be associated with acute exacerbations.

Obtain a social history
Document any recent drug or alcohol use. Cocaine use can cause acute chest pain.

Perform a general review of systems
This may help elicit any potential medical problems complicating the chest pain.

O — Perform a physical exam

Lungs: Note egophony, pleural rub, wheezing, or absent or decreased breath sounds.
Cardiac: Listen for murmurs, pericardial rub, irregular pulse, and S3 or S4 as signs of congestive heart failure.
Chest: Palpate the sternum, ribs, and chest wall for reproducible pain.
- Reproducible pain is more consistent with chest wall pain or costochondritis, but it does NOT exclude a myocardial infarction.

Extremities: Note pedal edema, pain with range of motion of arm/shoulders.

Check the ECG
If there are signs of a myocardial infarction (e.g., t-wave inversions, ST-segment elevation), see Myocardial Infarction p. 16.

Chest Pain

Obtain a CXR
Look for signs of infiltrate, pulmonary edema, pleural effusion, fractured ribs, or masses.

Check oxygen saturation
Low oxygen saturation on room air suggests pulmonary embolism, pulmonary edema, or pneumonia.

If there are multiple risk factors and/or an abnormal ECG, check cardiac enzymes
Approximately 10% to 25% of pts presenting to the ED can have a nondiagnostic ECG despite having a myocardial infarction.

A Musculoskeletal Chest Wall Pain   -or-   Pleurisy
Inflammation of the pleura, usually occurring as a complication of a disease (e.g., pneumonia, viral illness)

Costochondritis
Anterior chest wall pain caused by an irritated joint between the rib and the sternum

Differential Diagnosis
- Myocardial infarction
- Pneumonia
- Pneumothorax
- GERD/esophageal spasm
- Pulmonary embolism
- Aortic dissection

P Provide effective pain relief
NSAIDs work well on pain and the inflammatory response.
Narcotics pain relievers may be needed initially to control symptoms.

Encourage coughing and deep breathing exercises
Prevents atelectasis and secondary pneumonia when pts are splinting.

Musculoskeletal pain may respond to heat and stretching exercises

Educate pt
On the diagnosis and expected duration of illness

Ensure adequate follow-up with their primary care provider in the next week

Instruct pt to return to the ED for
Increased shortness of breath or chest pain
Fever greater than 102°F
Any other concerns or complaints

Congestive Heart Failure

S — What are the pt's current symptoms?
Common symptoms are:
- Shortness of breath
- Chest pain
- Orthopnea
- Palpitations
- Peripheral edema
- Generalized weakness or fatigue
- Dyspnea on exertion
- Racing heart beat

Have the symptoms developed gradually, or was there an abrupt onset?
Abrupt onset is seen with new-onset arrhythmias, myocardial infarction (MI), or acute onset of valvular heart disease (e.g., mitral regurgitation).
Gradual onset is seen with dietary indiscretion, noncompliance with medication, worsening of heart function, or renal insufficiency.

Does the pt have a history of congestive heart failure (CHF)?
If this is the initial presentation, need to exclude MI, myocarditis, pulmonary embolism (PE), hyperthyroidism, or new-onset valvular heart disease as a cause.

Obtain a thorough past medical history
Is there a history of MI, valvular heart disease, cardiomyopathy, hypertension, or diabetes?
- All are associated with CHF.

Is there a history of renal insufficiency?
- Can lead to fluid retention and secondary CHF.

Has the pt had any dietary indiscretions?
Noncompliance with a low-salt diet can trigger an exacerbation.

Obtain a medication list
Determine if the pt has been compliant with medications.

Obtain a review of symptoms
Fever and cough may be present with pneumonia or myocarditis.
Weight loss, heat intolerance, and tremors suggest hyperthyroidism, which can lead to high-output cardiac failure.

O — Perform a physical exam
HEENT: Note jugular venous distention, which is elevated in CHF.
Lungs: Rales, accessory muscle use, or respiratory distress may be seen.
Cardiac: Listen for murmurs; S3, S4 are seen in CHF.
Abdomen: Ascites supports long-standing CHF or liver failure.
Extremities: Diminished pulses and/or peripheral edema may be seen.
Neurologic: Mental status changes may be seen with hypoperfusion.

Obtain a CXR
Evaluate for prominence of pulmonary vessels, pleural effusion, and cardiomegaly.

Obtain an ECG
Exclude an acute MI or ongoing ischemia.
Exclude an arrhythmia as the cause.

Check the following labs
Cardiac enzymes: 30% of individuals with a CHF exacerbation will have elevated enzymes.

β-type natriuretic peptide (BNP)
- BNP is a neuropeptide released by the ventricles in response to overdistention.
- Level < 100 essentially rules out CHF.
- BNP levels correlate with the degree of symptoms and prognosis.
- Level > 400 has better diagnostic accuracy than physical exam and CXR.

BUN, creatinine, electrolytes to exclude renal insufficiency and electrolyte disturbance.
CBC to exclude anemia and elevated WBC count.

Consider an emergent echocardiogram if concerned about acute valvular compromise or cardiac tamponade

Echocardiogram can evaluate wall motion and valvular function, along with providing an estimated ejection fraction. However, an ejection fraction does not correlate well with symptoms.

A Congestive Heart Failure
Differential Diagnosis includes

- Pneumonia
- Myocardial infarction
- Pulmonary embolism
- Thyrotoxicosis
- Renal failure

P Place the pt on oxygen

If pt continues to have respiratory distress, consider a trial of continuous positive airway pressure or intubation.

Improve cardiac function

Decrease preload by administering:
- Nitroglycerin
- Morphine
- Loop diuretic

Decrease afterload (e.g., lower vascular resistance):
- Nitroglycerin
- β-blockers or Ca channel blockers may be needed if there is diastolic dysfunction.

Consider dopamine or dobutamine for increased inotropic support

Dobutamine can cause hypotension in about one-third of people who receive it.

Consider emergent cardiac catherization or thrombolytics

If there is evidence of an MI

Consider starting an ACE inhibitor

Can help reduce preload and afterload.
Use with caution in initial presentation and titrate dose upward slowly.

Admit to monitored nursing floor or ICU
Consider discharge

On rare occasions, a pt may be discharged if symptoms are mild, are improved in the ED, and if close follow-up can be arranged.

Endocarditis

S **What are the pt's current symptoms?**
Common presenting symptoms include:
- Fever
- Malaise
- Sweats
- Myalgias
- Arthralgias
- Weight loss
- Shortness of breath
- Chest pain
- Rash

Common complications of endocarditis that pts may present with include:
- Cerebrovascular accident
- Renal failure
- Myocardial infarction
- Chest pain from pulmonary infarction

Does the pt have any risk factors for endocarditis?
Indwelling venous catheter
History of endocarditis
Poor dentition
Intravenous drug abuse (IVDA)
Diabetes
Recent surgical procedure
Valvular heart disease
- Mitral valve prolapse
- Bicuspid aortic valve
- Prosthetic heart valve

Has the pt been on antibiotics recently?
May affect sensitivity of blood cultures.

Obtain a good review of symptoms
May elicit other causes of fever and/or infection source.

O **Perform a physical exam**
Look for physical signs of endocarditis:
- *Osler's nodes*: Painful nodular lesions normally seen on the extremities.
- *Janeway lesions*: Painless micro-hemorrhages typically seen on the palms or soles of feet.
- *Splinter hemorrhages*: Micro-hemorrhages under fingernails or toenails.
- *Roth spots*: Retinal hemorrhages with central clearing.
- *Petechiae*: Can be seen on mucosal membranes, conjunctiva, and hard palate.
- New onset of a murmur

Obtain an ECG
A heart block may be seen with extension of the infection into the atrioventricular node. Ischemic changes can be seen if the vegetations embolize down a coronary artery.

Obtain a CXR
May demonstrate pulmonary infarctions or pneumonia.

Obtain blood cultures
Two to three sets taken over several hours maximizes isolation of the causative agent.

Obtain CBC, electrolytes, and renal function tests
An elevated WBC may be seen.
Anemia is associated with subacute endocarditis.
May see renal failure from embolization to renal arteries.

Consider an echocardiogram
Evaluates heart valves and may notice vegetations.

TTE may miss 20% of vegetations. Consider TEE if clinical suspicion is > 4%.

A ## Endocarditis -or-
Noninfective Endocarditis
Duke criteria is used to make diagnosis. Need two major *or* one major and two minor *or* five minor criteria to make diagnosis.
- Major Criteria
    - Positive blood culture for typical organisms (HACEK, viridans streptococci, *Streptococcus bovis*) in two different blood cultures
    - Evidence of endocardial involvement
        - Oscillating intracardiac mass on valve or supporting structures, in the path of regurgitant jets, or on implanted material in the absence of an alternative anatomic explanation, or
        - Abscess, or
        - New partial dehiscence of prosthetic valve
- Minor Criteria
    - Predisposition: Predisposing heart condition or IVDA
    - Fever: temperature > 38.0°C (100.4°F)
    - *Vascular phenomena*: Major arterial emboli, septic pulmonary infarcts, mycotic aneurysm, intracranial hemorrhage, conjunctival hemorrhages, and Janeway lesions
    - *Immunologic phenomena*: Glomerulonephritis, Osler's nodes, Roth spots, and rheumatoid factor
    - *Microbiologic evidence*: Positive blood culture but does not meet a major criterion, as noted above, or serologic evidence of active infection with organism consistent with infective endocarditis (IE).
    - *Echocardiographic findings*: Consistent with IE but does not meet a major criterion, as noted above.

Differential Diagnosis
Systemic vasculitits
Rheumatologic disease

P ## Start empiric antibiotics
Consider vancomycin, gentamicin, and rifampin.

Consider surgical intervention for
Signs of congestive heart failure or hemodynamic compromise caused by valvular heart disease
Evidence of paravalvular abscess
Progressive heart block
Persistent bacteremia despite appropriate antibiotics
Infection of a prosthetic heart valve

Admit to monitored nursing floor or ICU
Need to monitor for progressive heart block and hemodynamic instability.

S — What are the pt's current symptoms?
Most pts with hypertension (HTN) are asymptomatic.
Symptoms that correlate with end-organ damage:
- Neurologic symptoms
    - Headache
    - Seizure
    - Confusion
    - Focal deficits
    - Coma
- Cardiac symptoms
    - Chest pain
    - Palpitations
    - Congestive heart failure (CHF)
- Renal symptoms
    - Hematuria
    - Oliguria
    - Proteinuria

Does the pt have a history of HTN?
If this is an initial presentation, need to exclude secondary causes of hypertension:
- Pheochromocytoma
- Primary hyperaldosteronism
- Cocaine and illicit drug use
- Coarctation of the aorta
- Renal artery stenosis

What medications is the pt taking?
Inquire about herbal supplements, especially ephedra.
Has the pt missed any doses? Can see rebound HTN with missed doses of clonidine.

Obtain a detailed social history
Inquire about illicit drug use, alcohol use, and tobacco use.

Perform a review of symptoms
May suggest a secondary cause of HTN.

O — Perform a physical exam
Fundoscopic exam: Evaluate for retinal hemorrhage and papillary edema, signs of end-organ damage.
Lungs: May hear rales as a sign of CHF.
Cardiac:
- Evaluate point of maximum impulse for a prominent apical impulse.
- Palpate for right ventricle heave.
- Make note of any murmur or S4.

Abdomen: Listen for renal bruits, sign of renal artery stenosis.
Neurologic: Ensure that there are no focal deficits or signs of a cerebrovascular accident (CVA).

Obtain an ECG
Evaluate for cardiac ischemia.
May see left ventricular hypertrophy as a sign of long-standing HTN.

Consider CT scan of head if there are any neurologic signs
Rule out intracranial bleed (ICB) or subarachnoid hemorrhage (SAH).

Obtain electrolytes, renal function tests, cardiac enzymes, and urinalysis
Rule out renal insufficiency.
May see hematuria and proteinuria.
Cardiac enzymes may be elevated as a result of cardiac injury and strain.

Obtain a urine drug screen if drug abuse is suspected
Obtain a CXR
May see signs of pulmonary congestion and cardiomegaly.
Evaluate mediastinum as possible aortic dissection.

Cardiology — Hypertensive Crisis

A

Hypertension
If pt's blood pressure is elevated, but there is no evidence of end-organ damage

Hypertensive Urgency
Severe HTN where there is a pending risk for end-organ damage
Blood pressure needs to be lowered over the next 24 hours in order to prevent end-organ injury.

Hypertensive Crisis/Emergency
Severely elevated blood pressure with evidence of end-organ damage
Blood pressure needs to be lowered immediately in order to prevent continued end-organ damage

Differential Diagnosis
- Pheochromocytoma
- CVA
- Brain tumor
- Cocaine or amphetamine use
- Aortic dissection
- ICB or SAH

P

Control the blood pressure
If asymptomatic and pt has not taken his home medications, you can give his usual home dosing and follow closely.
If asymptomatic, can give oral medications. Consider:
- Clonidine
- Nitroglycerin
- β-blockers
- Hydralazine
- Ca channel blockers
- ACE-inhibitors

If there is evidence of end-organ damage, immediate control of blood pressure warrants starting an IV medication for titratable control.
- Common medications used include:
  - Nitroprusside
  - Esmolol
- Goal drop in blood pressure is 20% to 25% of starting blood pressure over the first 60 minutes.
- Because of compensatory measures in the brain and kidneys, dropping the blood pressure too quickly can lead to CVA and hypoperfusion of the kidneys.
- Place arterial line for accurate and constant blood pressure measurement.

Admit to ICU if there is evidence of end-organ damage
Admit to monitored nursing floor for hypertensive urgency
Discharge home
If pt is asymptomatic, responded to treatment in the ED, and will have close follow-up with a primary care provider in the a.m., you can discharge home.

S — Determine the PQRST of the pain. (See Chest Pain p. 8.)
When inquiring about pain, ask if pts are having any discomfort, because some pts will deny pain but report intense pressure or a discomfort in their chest.

Have they had similar pain in the past? Does the pain change with exertion or stress?
Suggests prior history of angina

Does the pt have any risk factors for myocardial infarction (MI)?
Risk factors include a history of cigarette smoking, hypercholesterolemia, hypertension, diabetes, obesity, prior MI, male gender, prior angioplasty or percutaneous coronary angioplasty (PTCA), or family history of MI.
Diabetics frequently present without typical signs and symptoms of MI, and typically will not experience pain.

Does the pt have any associated symptoms?
Diaphoresis, shortness of breath, nausea, or vomiting

Has any treatment been initiated before your evaluation?
Have paramedics given nitroglycerin? Was there any improvement with treatment rendered?
Has the pt received aspirin or take aspirin daily?
Has the pt tried self-treatment with antacids? Did it help?

Obtain a medication list
Inquire if any medications have been missed or if there have been any recent changes

Obtain a past medical history
Particular attention needs to be paid to any history of coronary artery bypass graft or PTCA.
- When, which vessels, and were there any complications post-procedure?

Has there been any recent cardiac catherization or stress testing?

O — Evaluate vital signs
Ensure that pt is hemodynamically stable.

Perform a physical exam
Cardiac: May hear an S3 or a new murmur.
Lungs: Typically normal exam. Listen for rales, egophony, or pleural rub, which suggests an alternative diagnosis.
Often, the exam is normal and not very informative.

Obtain an ECG within 10 minutes of arrival
ST elevation in two or more contiguous leads or new left bundle branch block warrants emergent revascularization.
May also see hyperacute T waves, inverted T waves, or ST depression (reciprocal changes).
Consider a right-side ECG if there are peripheral signs of heart failure.

Approximately 20% of initial ECGs do not show any ischemic changes. Serial ECGs may be needed.

Obtain cardiac enzymes
CK, CKMB, and Trop-I may be elevated as early as 4 hrs after the onset of pain.
- Trop-I can remain elevated for up to 2 wks.

Myoglobin may be elevated as early as 2 hrs but lacks significant specificity.

Trop-I is the most specific enzyme available.

Several sets of enzymes over an 8- to 12-hour period are needed to completely rule out MI.

Obtain a CXR
May exclude other causes of chest pain.

A ### Myocardial Infarction
Sudden interruption or insufficiency of the supply of blood to the heart

Differential Diagnosis
- Unstable Angina
- Chest Pain
- Congestive heart failure
- Pleurisy
- Pneumonia
- Gastroesophageal reflux disease

P ### Initiate anti-ischemia therapy immediately. Pts should receive
Aspirin: 325 mg or four 81-mg aspirins. If on chronic aspirin therapy, this does not need to be repeated.
- Administer clopidogrel if pt is aspirin intolerant or PTCA is planned.

Nitroglycerin: Sublingual tablets, topical paste, or IV formulations are available.
- Titrate nitroglycerin for pain relief while ensuring that SBP remains greater than 90.

Morphine: Provides pain relief, decreases the preload, and reduces the pt's anxiety. The resulting effect is a decrease in overall myocardial oxygen demand and decrease in myocardial ischemia.

Heparin: Unfractionated or low-molecular-weight heparin; helps prevent extension of the plaque.

β-blocker: Avoid if pt is hypotensive, bradycardic, or has severe lung disease.
- Decreases cardiac oxygen demand.
- Has been shown to improve mortality if given within 12 hrs.

Arrange for emergent revascularization
Primary PTCA has been associated with improved outcomes if done within 2 hrs.
- If pt is going for primary PTCA, consider giving clopidogrel and/or a glycoprotein IIb/IIIa. Shown to decrease the rate of premature closure of the PTCA site.

Thrombolytics should be given if pain has been present for < 12 hrs, and primary PTCA cannot be done within 2 hrs.
- Major contraindications to thrombolytic therapy include:
  - Active bleeding
  - Major surgery or trauma in the past 3 wks
  - Neurosurgery or stroke in the past 3 months
  - Prolonged (> 10 minutes) or traumatic CPR

Monitor for reperfusion arrhythmias
Typically occur within the first hour after revascularization. VTach and an accelerated idioventricular tachycardia are most common. May see sinus bradycardia or complete heart block.

Admit to coronary care unit

Palpitations — Cardiology

S

What symptoms did the pt experience?
Pts may complain of a racing heart beat or a feeling of their heart skipping a beat.

Was there associated lightheadedness or syncope?
Seen with arrhythmias that cause hemodynamic compromise. Requires a more thorough workup because it may be a warning sign for sudden cardiac death.

What was the pt doing when the palpitations started?
Exercise and psychological stress may induce arrhythmias.

Inquire about recent caffeine, alcohol, tobacco, or cocaine/amphetamine use
These agents can cause myocardial irritation and excitation, causing arrhythmias.

How long did the palpitations last, and are they still present?
Does the pt have a history of palpitations, coronary atherosclerotic disease (CAD), or congestive heart failure (CHF)?
Palpitations may be a sign of ischemia or CHF exacerbation.
If they have had palpitations before, do they know what arrhythmia they had and how it was treated? May help direct your current treatment.

What has the pt done to try and stop the palpitations?
Some pts know to try a valsalva maneuver (e.g., cough, carotid massage, or bearing down).

Obtain a thorough past medical history
History of chronic obstructive pulmonary disease (COPD) or pulmonary disorders are associated with atrial flutter, atrial fibrillation, and multifocal atrial tachycardia.
History of CHF or CAD is associated with VTach, heart blocks, and premature ventricular contractions (PVCs).

O

Perform a physical exam
Look for signs of a CHF or COPD exacerbation. Generally, the exam is normal and not very helpful in determining the cause of the arrhythmia.

Obtain an ECG. Look for signs of ischemia, heart block, or an arrhythmia.
Atrial flutter will show flutter waves, which are organized, rapid (300 bpm) depolarizations of the atrium with variable conduction to the ventricles.
Atrial fibrillation will have an absence of P waves because atrial activity is disorganized, with irregular conduction to the ventricles.
VTach will typically show a regular ventricular response with a widened QRS complex. Ventricular response is independent of any atrial activity.
Look for Delta waves: A shortened PR interval with a slurring of the initial portion of the QRS complex. Diagnostic of Wolfe-Parkinson-White syndrome and represents a bypass tract between the atrium and the ventricles.

Place pt on a cardiac monitor
Obtain a CXR. May show signs of pneumonia or CHF exacerbation.
Check electrolytes and/or thyroid-stimulating hormone (TSH)
Hypo-/hyperthyroidism and electrolyte imbalances of potassium, calcium, or magnesium may cause arrhythmias.

If suspicious for cardiac ischemia (e.g., chest pain), check cardiac enzymes

A **Atrial Fibrillation/Flutter** -or-
Supraventricular Tachycardia/PSVT -or-
Ventricular Tachycardia -or-
Premature Ventricular Contractions (PVCs)

P **Consider an adenosine challenge**
If unable to determine rhythm because of a rapid rate, consider an adenosine challenge. Administer 6, 12, or 18 mg of adenosine rapid IV push. Causes transient block of the atrioventricular (AV) node, allowing you to see the atrial activity. Can be associated with a brief period of asystole.
May correct palpitations caused by AV nodal reentrant tachycardia.

Consider cardioversion
If pt becomes hemodynamically unstable as per advanced cardiac life support (ACLS) protocols

Premature ventricular contractions do not require any treatment if there is no evidence of hemodynamic compromise
If pt had lightheadedness or syncope, need to rule out undiagnosed VTach.

Atrial fibrillation/flutter
Typically require admission to a monitored nursing floor (MNF) for anticoagulation and workup to consist of TSH and echocardiogram.
Cardioversion should not be attempted in the ED until after the pt has been fully evaluated because of the risk of CVA.
Treat any underlying pulmonary disorder that may be exacerbating the cardiac arrhythmia.
Control rate with calcium channel blockers, β-blockers, and/or digoxin.
If concerned about Wolff-Parkinson-White syndrome, rate can be controlled with procainamide. Avoid digoxin, calcium channel blockers, and β-blockers.

Supraventricular Tachycardia/PSVT
May be associated with tobacco, alcohol, caffeine, and drug use.
Typically transient in nature, and treatment is to discontinue the causative agent.
Can obtain rate control with β-blockers, calcium channel blockers.
If recurrent or evidence of an accessory pathway, pt may require an electrophysiology (EP) study.

Ventricular Tachycardia
If stable, can attempt to convert by administering lidocaine or amiodarone.
- Amiodarone will affect your ability to perform an EP study, although it is considered the first-line agent according to ACLS protocols.

Admit to MNF or ICU
Consider discharge home
If pt's symptoms were mild, workup in ED was negative, and there is good follow-up, consider sending the pt home with a Holter monitor.

S — Did the pt truly lose consciousness? Was the event witnessed?
If witnessed, determine how long the pt was unconscious and if there were any symptoms leading up to the event.
Ask about seizure activity or incontinence.
- Some pts can have jerking movement of their limbs that are believed to be seizures by the lay bystander.

How long did it take for the pt to begin to think and act normally?
- Syncope should have a quick return to baseline, where a seizure may have a prolonged postictal phase.

What was the pt doing before the syncopal episode?
Prolonged standing, standing up quickly, and emotional upset can all trigger a vasovagal episode, leading to syncope.
Defecating and micturition can trigger a syncopal episode by activating hypersensitive peripheral receptors.

Has the pt been eating or drinking appropriately?
Does the pt have a history of syncope?
Determine circumstances around prior episodes. Has the pt had any testing done to determine the etiology?

Where there any symptoms before the episode?
Lightheadedness, chest pain, palpitations, and a racing heart beat all suggest a cardiac cause of syncope.
Headache, confusion, focal weakness, or numbness suggests a neurologic cause.

Does the pt have a history of diabetes, seizures, coronary atherosclerotic disease, hypertension, congestive heart failure, or arrhythmias?
Prior cardiac history increases risk for myocardial infarction (MI) and arrhythmias.

Is there a history of hypoglycemia?
Has the pt started any new medications? What medications are being taken?
New hypertensive agents may be causing postural hypotension and syncope.

O — Evaluate the pt's vital signs
Perform orthostatics, which will help determine if postural hypotension is the cause.

Perform a physical exam
Look for signs of trauma or injury.
Evaluate mental status, and ensure that there are no neurologic deficits.
Perform a rectal exam to rule out occult GI bleeding.
Generally, the physical exam is completely normal.

Obtain an ECG
Evaluate for ischemia or signs of arrhythmia.

Check the pt's blood sugar
New-onset diabetes with dehydration may present with syncope.

Cardiology — Syncope

If history suggests or pt has risk factors for MI, obtain cardiac enzymes
If there were any neurologic symptoms preceding the event, obtain a CT scan of the head
Exclude intracranial bleed, subarachnoid hemorrhage, or space-occupying mass as cause.
Consider a CT if the pt has fallen and there is evidence of a head injury.

If there is a possibility of pregnancy, check β-hCG
If pt has a seizure disorder, considering checking levels of any antiseizure medications

A **Syncope**
In most cases, a cause for the syncopal episode cannot be determined. A good history is your best weapon in determining the cause.
- Most clinical studies are normal and nondiagnostic.

Differential Diagnosis
- Seizure
- Cerebrovascular accident
- Hypoglycemia
- Anxiety or panic attack

P **Treat hypoglycemia with intravenous fluids (IVFs) and D50.** (See Hypoglycemia p. 38.)
Treat arrhythmias as indicated
If orthostatic or signs of dehydration present, administer IVFs
Recheck orthostatics after fluid resuscitation to ensure that symptoms have resolved.

If pt has suffered an injury, further inpatient workup is warranted
Generally, suggests that there was no warning or preceding symptoms that indicated a sudden cardiac arrhythmia as cause.

Consider obtaining an echocardiogram, if valvular heart disease is suspected.
Admit pts to a monitored nursing floor or the ICU with any of the following
- Syncope while supine
- Old age
- Trauma
- Recurrent syncope
- Prolonged loss of consciousness
- Headache or focal neurologic signs
- Young pt with exertional syncope

Consider discharge home
Pts that have classic vasovagal syncope where the precipitating factor is identified (e.g., prolonged standing in church) and no cardiac symptoms or significant risk factors can be discharged home.

22 Unstable Angina — Cardiology

S

Determine the PQRST of the pain. (See Chest Pain p. 8.)

Does the pt have a known history of angina?
Has there been a change in the amount of exercise the pt can perform before getting short of breath or developing chest pain?
Has the pt experienced chest pain at rest?
All initial diagnoses of angina are considered unstable by definition.

Do any specific actions exacerbate the chest pain?
Walking, stair climbing, or aerobic exercise is more consistent with cardiac ischemia.

What makes the pain or symptoms resolve?
Pain that resolves quickly with rest or nitroglycerin is consistent with angina.
Nitroglycerin can relieve esophageal pain and spasm; therefore, relief with nitroglycerin is not diagnostic of angina.

Does the pt have any associated symptoms?
Shortness of breath, nausea, vomiting, and diaphoresis. Diaphoresis is not a common symptom and should increase your suspicion for true pain/ischemia.

Has the pt undergone any coronary revascularization procedures in the past?
Symptoms following coronary artery bypass graft (CABG) or percutaneous coronary angioplasty (PTCA) can be caused by subacute closure of the grafts or angioplasty site.

What are the pt's risk factors for coronary atherosclerosis?
See Myocardial Infarction p. 16.

Ask about any new medications or whether the pt has missed any doses
Recurrence of angina may be caused by pt noncompliance with medical management.

Perform a general review of systems
This may help elicit any potential medical problems complicating the chest pain.

O

Perform a physical exam
Lungs: Typically normal, may hear rales or wheezing if congestive heart failure (CHF) present.
Chest: Note any reproducible pain, although it may be present with cardiac ischemia.
Cardiac: Note any irregular pulse, murmurs, S3 or S4.
Extremities: Note any pedal edema, seen with CHF.
Rectal exam: Must be performed to rule out occult GI bleeding if you plan to initiate anticoagulation therapy.

Check the ECG
Be sure to compare it to an old ECG. Occasionally, individuals will demonstrate pseudo-normalization (e.g., their baseline T-waves are inverted, but now they are upright and normal-appearing on your present ECG) of their ECG, making it difficult to diagnose ischemia changes.

Obtain a CXR
Look for signs of infiltrate, pulmonary edema, pleural effusion, cardiomegaly, or widened mediastinum (suggest aortic dissection).

Check the following labs
Cardiac enzymes
- Myoglobin will show elevations within 2 hrs, although it is not specific for cardiac injury.
- Elevation in Trop-I is diagnostic of cardiac muscle injury.
- Elevation in CK can be seen with any muscle injury.
- Individuals with renal failure may have chronically elevated CK, CKMB.
- NQWMI or non-ST elevation myocardial infarction can only be ruled out by obtaining serial enzymes over a 6- to 12-hr period.

Electroytes, BUN, Creatinine: Rule out electrolyte disturbance or renal failure.
CBC: Ensure that anemia is not the cause of ischemia.

A ### Unstable Angina
Severe paroxysmal pain in the chest associated with an insufficient supply of blood to the heart that is occurring at rest or with increasing frequency. Pain should be relieved with rest or nitroglycerin.

Myocardial Infarction
Sudden interruption or insufficiency of the supply of blood to the heart

Differential Diagnosis
- Chest pain   - Pneumonia   - Pulmonary embolism

P ### Initiate treatment for ischemia
Institute the following treatment:
- Place pt on oxygen.
- Give nitroglycerin sublingually or IV if SBP > 100.
- Give aspirin 325 mg if not allergic.
- Consider administering β-blocker if heart rate > 70.
- Consider morphine 2 to 4 mg IV as needed for pain.

If pt has ECG changes, consider starting heparin therapy.

Titrate medications to provide effective pain relief
Ongoing pain represents continued cardiac muscle injury.

If the pt has ECG changes or has had a recent PTCA or CABG, discuss the case with the pt's cardiologist or primary care provider
Discuss initiating glycoprotein IIb/IIIa therapy if pt has ST depression, positive cardiac enzymes, high risk for ischemia, or if emergency revascularization is planned.

Arrange admission to a monitored nursing floor or coronary care unit

S — Does the pt have pain or swelling in one or both legs?
Deep venous thrombosis (DVT) may involve both legs, but typically is found in only one leg.
Bilateral swelling is more consistent with congestive heart failure (CHF).

Does the pt have any risk factors for a venous thrombosis?
Risk factors include the following:
- Recent surgery or immobilization
- Estrogen or birth control pill use
- Pregnancy
- History of hypercoagulable state
- Tobacco use
- Recent travel
- Cancer
- Prior history of DVT/pulmonary embolism (PE)

Does the pt have any associated symptoms of chest pain or shortness of breath?
May signify a PE and warrants additional evaluation.

Has the pt suffered any trauma to the extremity?
Suggests pain and swelling caused by cellulites or focal abscess.
Recent fracture increases the risk for DVT.

Obtain a thorough past medical history
History of cirrhosis, renal insufficiency, or CHF may explain swelling in lower extremities.
Prior surgery or saphenous vein graft harvest for coronary artery bypass graft are associated with chronic leg swelling postoperatively.

Has the pt been placed on any new medications or have any medications been discontinued?
Any change in CHF or cirrhosis management may lead to increased peripheral edema.

O — Perform a physical exam
Lungs: Listen for pleural rub, which may be seen with PE.
Cardiac: Listen for new murmurs and palpate for right ventricle heave, which may occur with PE.
Extremities: Measure both calves and compare, palpate for venous cords.
- Are there any signs of cellulitis (e.g., redness, warmth, swelling, tenderness)?

Check the following labs
CBC, coagulation studies: Baseline studies in case anticoagulation is needed.
Consider checking a D-dimer: ELISA D-dimer is 80% sensitive but nonspecific for DVT.
Consider performing a hypercoagulable evaluation.
- Important to consider in the ED because testing can be affected by the start of heparin and/or warfarin therapies.

Obtain duplex venous Dopplers
High sensitivity/specificity for proximal veins, but less so for distal calf veins. Test performance is affected by body habitus and tissue edema.
May see Baker's cyst as cause of swelling.
Cannot evaluate pelvic veins.

Consider MRI
If there is a strong suspicion for pelvic or inferior vena cava (IVC) thrombosis, which is common after Ob/Gyn surgery.

Consider PE evaluation if pt has chest pain or shortness of breath
See Pulmonary Embolism p. 54.

A

Deep Venous Thrombosis
A blood clot in the deep veins of the legs. Blood clots above the knee have an increased risk of dislodging and becoming a PE.

Superficial Venous Thrombosis
A blood clot in the superficial veins of the legs not associated with PE

Differential Diagnosis
- Cellulitis
- CHF
- Lymphedema
- Cirrhosis
- Nephrotic syndrome

P

Deep Venous Thrombosis
Begin anticoagulation to prevent clot propagation and PE if no risk factors exist.
- Risk factors include:
  - Recent intracranial bleed or subarachnoid hemorrhage
  - Active gastrointestinal bleeding
  - High risk for falls and subsequent head injury
- Low-molecular-weight heparin or unfractionated heparin can be initiated.
  - Can discontinue heparin therapy once warfarin has been therapeutic for 2 days.
- Warfarin therapy will be needed for 6 months.
  - If second DVT/PE or hypercoagulable state is found, pt will need lifelong warfarin therapy.

Consider IVC filter placement in pts:
- Not suitable for anticoagulation
- Who developed DVT or PE while on anticoagulation
- With tenuous respiratory status where any PE may result in death

Treat pain with NSAIDs or narcotic pain relievers.

Superficial Venous Thrombosis
No indication for anticoagulation therapy unless clot is propagating into deep system.
Initiate conservative therapy.
- Rest
- Elevation
- Warm compresses
- NSAIDs

II
Hematology

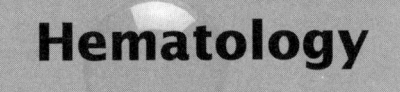

Anemia

S **Is the pt symptomatic?**
Most anemias are picked up by routine testing and pts are completely asymptomatic. A hemoglobin (Hb) < 12 mg/dL indicates anemia.

Does the pt have a history of blood in the stool or black, tarry stools?
A sign of gastrointestinal blood loss and a leading cause of anemia

Has the pt experienced any fatigue, exertional dyspnea, or chest pain?
These are common symptoms of anemia.
Other symptoms include:
- Cold intolerance
- Altered mental status or ability to concentrate
- Postural hypotension or syncope
- Headaches
- Decreased exercise tolerance

Does the pt have a history of heavy menstrual bleeding?
Has the pt been a victim of a recent trauma?
Occult internal injuries will need to be ruled out.

If a child, inquire about lead in the home and whether the child has undergone lead testing
More common with inner-city children.

Obtain a detailed past medical history
Chronic medical conditions can lead to anemia:
- Cancer
- Cirrhosis
- Congestive heart failure
- Lupus
- Renal failure
- Hypothyroidism

History of gastric or intestinal surgery can lead to pernicious anemia.

Is the pt taking any medications or herbal supplements?
Many medications can cause bone marrow suppression and/or increased destruction of red blood cells.

Does the pt have a history of alcohol abuse?
Alcohol has a direct toxic effect on the bone marrow and increases the risk for GI bleeding.

Obtain a thorough review of symptoms
May find symptoms of infection or easy bruising, which suggest a diagnosis of thrombotic thrombocytopenic purpura (TTP) or disseminated intravascular coagulation (DIC).

O **Perform a physical exam**
Typically, the exam will be normal.
Look for petechiae or purpura as signs of idiopathic thrombocytopenic purpura (ITP)/TTP.
Pale conjunctiva and pale palmar creases signify significant blood loss.
Tachycardia may be seen with acute blood loss.
Scleral icterus and jaundice may be seen with hemolysis.
Glossitis, loss of the papillae on the tongue, can be seen in iron-deficiency anemia and pernicious anemia.
Perform rectal exam to evaluate for occult blood loss.

Obtain the following labs
CBC:
- Hb < 12 confirms the diagnosis.
- The mean corpuscular volume will help differentiate the anemia as microcytic (< 80) or macrocytic (> 100).
  - Microcytic anemia is seen in iron-deficiency anemia and anemia of chronic disease.
  - Macrocytic anemia is seen in folate and B_{12} deficiency.
- Note any schistocytes, which can be seen with intravascular hemolysis.
- Thrombocytopenia may signify DIC, ITP, or TTP.

Liver function tests, reticulocyte count, haptoglobin, and lactate dehydrogenase (LDH):
- Hemolysis will have ↑ reticulocyte count, LDH, and bilirubin and ↓ haptoglobin.
- Bone marrow failure will have an inappropriately low reticulocyte count.

Iron studies (total iron-binding capacity [TIBC], ferritin, transferrin, iron level) if iron deficiency is suspected
- ↓ ferritin, reticulocyte count, and iron level with ↓ TIBC is seen.
- May need bone marrow biopsy to fully evaluate iron stores.

B_{12} and folate levels if macrocytic anemia is noted.
- Important to check B_{12} deficiency because treatment with folate can correct the anemia, but persistent B_{12} deficiency can lead to neurologic complications.

Renal function tests to exclude renal failure as cause of the anemia.

A Anemia of Chronic Disease -or-
Iron-Deficiency Anemia -or-
Folate/B_{12}-Deficiency Anemia
Differential Diagnosis
Disseminated intravascular coagulation (DIC)
Idiopathic thrombocytopenic purpura (ITP)
Thrombotic thrombocytopenic purpura (TTP)
Renal failure
Gastrointestinal bleeding

P Provide IV fluids and place on oxygen if symptomatic
Type and cross for packed red blood cells
Transfuse if Hb < 10 and pt is symptomatic or has history of ischemic heart disease. Otherwise, there is no indication to transfuse unless Hb < 7.

Consider GI evaluation
If rectal exam revealed guaiac-positive stool or frank blood.

Supplement iron, B_{12}, and folate as required
Discharge if
- Asymptomatic
- No signs of active blood loss
- Most pts will be able to be discharged.
- Hb > 8
- Close follow-up is arranged

Admit if
- Symptomatic
- Active blood loss
- Initial Hb < 8
- Significant comorbid conditions

S Has the pt noticed any unusual bleeding or bruising?
Thrombotic thrombocytopenic purpura (TTP) and idiopathic thrombocytopenic purpura (ITP) are associated with:
- Easy bruising
- Petechiae/purpura
- GI bleeding
- Epistaxis
- Gingival bleeding
- Menorrhagia

Is there any history of fever, headache, confusion, or hematuria?
TTP is a pentad of:
- Thrombocytopenia
- Microangiopathic hemolytic anemia
- Neurologic signs and symptoms
- Renal dysfunction
- Fever

Has the pt suffered from a recent viral illness?
ITP is associated with viral prodrome.

Does the pt have a history of TTP/ITP?
With current treatment, pts may go into remission and have an acute exacerbation at a later time.

Has the pt been started on any new medications or herbal supplements?
TTP may be triggered by medications, infection, and pregnancy.

Obtain a detailed medical history
May help determine a possible causative agent. TTP is associated with autoimmune disorders.

Conduct a thorough review of symptoms
GI bleeding, cardiac ischemia, and shortness of breath may all occur as a result of the anemia or thrombosis associated with TTP.

O Perform physical exam
Skin: Look for petechiae or purpura.
HEENT: Note any gingival bleeding, mucosal petechiae, or epistaxis.
Abdomen: Palpate the liver and spleen carefully and note any organomegaly.
Rectal exam: Exclude GI blood loss.
Neurologic: May have mental status changes or focal deficits.

Obtain the following labs
CBC to check for anemia and thrombocytopenia.
- Check smear for schistocytes (sign of intravascular hemolysis and TTP).

Liver function tests, lactate dehydrogenase, haptoglobin as indicators of hemolysis.
BUN, Creatinine to exclude renal failure.
β-hCG to exclude pregnancy.
Coagulation studies to exclude other bleeding diathesis.
Urinalysis: May see proteinuria or hematuria as signs of renal failure, exclude urinary tract infection as inciting event.
Blood cultures to exclude occult bacteremia as inciting event.

If neurologic symptoms present, obtain a head CT scan
Exclude cerebrovascular accident (CVA), intracranial bleed, subarachnoid hemorrhage.

Hematology

Consider abdominal CT to evaluate degree of hypersplenism

A **Thrombotic Thrombocytopenic Purpura**
Thrombocytopenia is caused by diffuse vessel wall injury that leads to microangiopathic hemolytic anemia and consumption of platelets. Secondary organ injury (renal failure, central nervous system symptoms) occurs from thrombosis formation at the site of wall injury.

-or-

Idiopathic Thrombocytopenic Purpura
Platelet destruction is caused by antiplatelet antibodies that are often associated with a viral illness.
An auto-immune disease

Differential Diagnosis
- Disseminated intravascular coagulation (DIC)
- HELLP
- Viral infection
- Leukemia/lymphoma

P **If diagnosis remains vague**
Consult Hematology/Oncology ASAP.
Consider scheduling for bone marrow biopsy ASAP.

Admit all cases of DIC and TTP
May discharge pt with ITP if
- No significant bleeding
- Platelets > 30,000
- Close follow-up can be arranged

Thrombotic Thrombocytopenic Purpura
Plasma exchange is the treatment of choice.
Intravenous immunoglobulin (IVIG) may play a role.
Do NOT transfuse platelets except in cases of life-threatening bleeding.
- Platelet transfusion can increase thrombosis formation, leading to CVA, renal failure, and myocardial infarction.

Idiopathic Thrombocytopenic Purpura
Self-limited in children, but may be persistent and chronic in adults with frequent exacerbations.
Steroids are the mainstay of treatment.
IVIG may play a role.
Splenectomy may be needed for refractory cases.
Immunosuppressive and chemotherapeutic agents have been used to achieve remission.
If asymptomatic, some pts can be followed closely and no treatment is needed.

Sickle Cell Disease

S **What is the pt's main complaint?**
Symptoms of sickle cell disease (SCD) can be divided into six physiologic areas:
- *Anemia*: pallor and fatigue
- *Hemolysis*: jaundice and cholelithiasis
- *Vaso-occlusive crisis*: pain in back, chest, or abdomen
- *Acute chest syndrome*: severe pleuritic chest pain, hypoxemia, tachypnea, and dyspnea
- *Splenic sequestration*: splenomegaly, fever, abdominal pain
- *Aplastic crisis*: rapid onset of profound anemia usually triggered by an infection

Does the pt have a history of sickle cell trait or sickle cell anemia?
Sickle cell trait pts tend to have less severe symptoms and complications.

Could anything have triggered this crisis?
Common inciting events to trigger a sickle cell crisis are:

- Fever	- Infection	- Stress
- Pregnancy	- Hypoxemia	- Alcohol
- Menstruation	- Dehydration	- Temperature changes

Has the pt been immunized against *Streptococcus pneumonias* and *Haemophilus influenzae*?
Functional asplenia in SCD leaves pts vulnerable to infections with encapsulated organisms.

Obtain a past medical history
Has the pt received blood transfusions in the past?
Have there been any major complications from SCD, such as acute chest syndrome, cerebrovascular accident (CVA), renal insufficiency, osteomyelitis, or avascular necrosis of the hip?
Are there any other comorbid diseases such as diabetes and/or hypertension?

Obtain a medication list
Current therapies include hydroxyurea and erythropoietin.
Does the pt take narcotics for chronic pain? Will help guide how much pain medicine to give in the ED.

O **Perform a physical exam**
Lungs: Listen for egophony and wheezing as signs of pneumonia. Pleural rub may be heard with pleural infarctions.
Cardiac: Note any murmurs.
Abdomen: Spleen is generally only palpable in young pts or those with splenic sequestration.
Extremities: May have leg ulcers, pain with range of motion, or finger swelling.
Neurologic: May have focal deficits with CVA.
Skin: Note any pallor or jaundice, signs of cellulitis.

Obtain the following labs
CBC:
- Evaluate degree of anemia, may see sickle cells on smear.
  - Compare Hb to prior labs to see if there has been any significant change.
- Elevated WBC can be seen with infection or crisis.

Reticulocyte count: Should be elevated. Decreased during aplastic or hypoplastic crisis.
LFT: Bilirubin elevated with hemolysis.

BUN, creatinine: Elevated in renal failure that may be caused by hypoperfusion or renal infarcts.
Blood cultures, urinalysis, and urine culture to rule out infection.
Type and cross

Perform lumbar puncture if meningitis is suspected
SCD pts can succumb in hours if infected with an encapsulated organism.

Check CXR
Excludes pneumonia or pulmonary infarcts.

Obtain head CT if any neurologic symptoms are present
Exclude hemorrhagic CVA, intracranial bleed, or subarachnoid hemorrhage from differential.

Consider x-rays of any painful limbs
Exclude occult fracture, osteomyelitis, or osteonecrosis from the differential.

A Sickle Cell Crisis
Diagnosis is usually well-established before presentation.

Differential Diagnosis for new onset
- Iron-deficiency anemia   - Thalassemia   - Leukemia

P **Start oxygen therapy.** Maintain SpO_2 > 92% to prevent peripheral sickling.
Provide aggressive IV hydration with normal saline solution initially

Once euvolemic, start D5 1/2 NS because of hyposthenuria (inability to form urine of high specific gravity common in SCD).

Treat pain with IV narcotics
Meperidine is discouraged (more addictive and increased risk of seizures at high doses). Morphine is drug of choice. Consider a patient-controlled analgesia pump.

Transfuse packed red blood cells for
- Hb < 5   - Symptomatic anemia   - Splenic sequestration
- Acute chest syndrome   - Aplastic anemia   crisis

Do not transfuse if Hb > 8 because may worsen symptoms caused by increased blood viscosity.

Start antibiotics immediately
If pt has fever or you suspect an infection
Susceptible to overwhelming infection with high mortality if not treated aggressively.

Consider starting hydroxyurea
Increases production of fetal hemoglobin to augment O_2 delivery.

Arrange for admission
Only those pts with mild pain that quickly corrects with IV narcotics should be considered for discharge with close follow-up.

III
Endocrine

Diabetic Ketoacidosis

S **Does the pt have a history of diabetes?**
Diabetic ketoacidosis (DKA) is the presenting diagnosis in approximately 20% of newly diagnosed diabetics.
Has the pt neglected to take insulin? Missing even one dose of insulin can cause an episode of DKA. Typically, pts will not eat if they feel sick, and thinking that it will cause hypoglycemia, they do not take their insulin.
Nonketotic hyperglycemia (NKH) typically occurs in elderly people who have renal impairment or decreased thirst response.

What are the pt's current symptoms?
Common symptoms in DKA are:
- Polyuria
- Polydipsia
- Lightheadedness
- Fatigue
- Nausea/vomiting
- Blurred vision
- Generalized weakness
- Mental status changes
- Abdominal pain
- Acetone breath
- Kussmaul respirations

NKH presents with similar symptoms except abdominal pain, respiration abnormalities, or acetone breath because there is no ketone production.

Does the pt have any symptoms of an infection?
An infection can trigger an episode of DKA or NKH.

What medications is the pt taking?
Steroids may cause DKA or NKH.
Isoniazid, iron, and salicylate (aspirin) overdose can mimic the signs/symptoms of DKA.

Could any stressors have triggered this episode? Common triggers include:
- Recent surgery or trauma
- Myocardial infarction
- Hyperthyroidism
- Cerebrovascular accident
- Pancreatitis
- Stress

Does the pt have any major medical problems?
Identify any comorbid conditions.

O **Perform a physical exam**
HEENT: Note appearance of mucous membranes.
Lungs: Listen for signs of pneumonia or bronchitis.
Skin: Note any signs of cellulitis or infection. Note any decreased skin turgor.

Obtain the following labs
CBC: May reveal leukocytosis as evidence of infection and/or ketosis.
Electrolytes: Calculate anion gap. Typically > 12 in DKA because of the metabolic acidosis.

- Pseudo-hyponatremia caused by hyperglycemia may be noted. Na = Na + 2*((Glucose − 100)/100)

BUN, Creatinine: May be elevated as a result of dehydration and prerenal azotemia.
Glucose: Glucose in NKH is typically 1000–1500, in DKA < 800.
Potassium, magnesium, phosphorus: Follow closely because they will probably all require replacement.
Urinalysis: Look for source of infection; note ketones and glucosuria.
ABG: Evaluate degree of metabolic acidosis.
β-hydroxybutyrate: Ketoacidosis is seen in DKA. Mild ketoacidosis may be seen in NKH.

Endocrine — Diabetic Ketoacidosis

If infection is suspected, obtain (e.g., cough, fever, dysuria):
- CXR
- Blood cultures × 2
- Urine culture

If possible toxic ingestion is suspected
Obtain serum osmolarity and calculate osmolar gap.

- Calculated serum osmolarity = 2*Na + Glu/18 + BUN/2.8 + EtOH/4.6
- Gap should be approximately 10. If > 10, suspect toxic ingestion.

Check Tylenol, ethanol (EtOH), and salicylate levels.

A

Diabetic Ketoacidosis
Hyperglycemic state characterized by metabolic acidosis and ketone production
Commonly seen in insulin-dependent diabetics

Nonketotic hyperosmolar coma
Hyperglycemic state characterized by mental status changes without significant ketone production. Commonly occurs in non-insulin-dependent diabetics.

Differential Diagnosis
- Overdose
- EtOH intoxication
- Sepsis

P

Start aggressive hydration with normal saline solution
May have fluid deficit of 5–10 L. Give 1–2 L bolus and replete remainder over 12 hrs. Hydration alone will help lower glucose level through renal excretion.

Replace electrolytes as needed
Most pts tend to be whole body depleted in potassium, magnesium, and phosphorus.
Need to replace magnesium before potassium replacement.
Potassium level may initially appear normal, although it will drop once acidosis is corrected.

Start insulin therapy
Administer an IV bolus followed by an insulin infusion. Avoid bolus in young children because of risk of cerebral edema with too rapid a correction in the glucose level.
- For DKA, start insulin infusion at 0.05–0.1 units/kg/hr.
- For NKA, start insulin infusion at half DKA rates.

Avoid subcutaneous insulin because its absorption is sporadic and its half-life is too long to allow tight control of glucose initially.
Continue insulin infusion until the acidosis is corrected regardless of the glucose level.
Add dextrose to IVF if glucose < 250 to prevent hypoglycemia.

Consider bicarbonate infusion
Bicarbonate infusion should be restricted to only extreme acidosis with evidence of cardiovascular collapse because it may actually increase intracellular acidosis and further exacerbate hypokalemia.

Treat any infections that are found
Arrange for admission

S What are the pt's current symptoms?
Common symptoms include:
- Tachycardia
- Anxiety
- Headache
- Diaphoresis
- Hyperventilation
- Mental status changes or coma
- Convulsions

Does the pt have a history of hypoglycemia?
Reactive hypoglycemia typically occurs 2 to 4 hrs after meals because of an exaggerated or delayed release of insulin. Associated with a progression to type II diabetes.

Does the pt have a history of diabetes?
Insulin overdose and sulfonylurea use can both cause hypoglycemia.

Does the pt have a history of or symptoms of renal failure?
Insulin's half-life is increased in renal failure, which may lead to higher circulating levels.

Does the pt take any medications or herbal supplements?
Sulfonylureas and fluoroquinolones, especially in combination, have been associated with profound hypoglycemia.
A single glipizide tablet can be fatal in a young child.

Has the pt been fasting?
Is there any history of endocrine disorders?
Pituitary insufficiency, adrenal insufficiency, and hypothyroidism have all been associated with hypoglycemia.

Is there a history of alcohol abuse or pancreatitis?
Alcohol consumption may cause pancreatitis.
Chronic pancreatitis can affect the endocrine function of the pancreas, leading to hypoglycemia.

Is there a history of depression or excessive weight loss?
Both are associated with factitious insulin administration and hypoglycemia.

Does the pt have any other medical problems?

O Perform a physical exam
Typically normal except for mental status changes and possible coma.

Check pt's blood sugar with a glucometer
Easy bedside test that can provide diagnosis within seconds. It is imperative that the diagnosis is made quickly and the hypoglycemia corrected because pt can suffer irreparable neurologic damage.
If unable to obtain bedside blood sugar, err on the side of caution and administer D50.

Obtain the following labs
CBC, electrolytes, BUN, and creatinine: Exclude anemia, electrolyte disturbance, or renal failure as possible causes.
Glucose, insulin, and C-peptide levels: An elevated insulin level will be seen in pts with an exogenous administration of insulin or an insulinoma. The C-peptide level may be helpful when attempting to distinguish between these two diagnoses. The C-peptide level is only elevated by the endogenous production of insulin. Therefore, it will be low or normal in exogenous administration.

Consider thyroid-stimulating hormone, cortisol levels
If hypo-/hyperthyroidism or adrenal insufficiency is suspected

Consider ethanol level and drug screen
If pt does not improve quickly with glucose administration or etiology of symptoms is unclear

Obtain head CT scan
If mental status does not return to normal with glucose administration

Consider lumbar puncture if encephalitis or meningitis is suspected

A

Hypoglycemia
Whipple's triad: (1) Symptoms consistent with hypoglycemia, (2) low glucose, and (3) resolution of symptoms with correction of glucose.

Differential Diagnosis of decreased mental status/coma includes
- Alcohol intoxication
- Drug overdose
- Cerebrovascular accident
- Meningitis/Encephalitis
- Depression/Psychosis
- Infection

P

Administer 1 amp of dextrose 50% ASAP
Any delay may cause additional irreparable neurologic damage.

Consider Glucagon
If dextrose 50% is not available or IV access is unobtainable:
Administer IM glucagon. Increases glucose release from the liver.

If hypoglycemia is caused by sulfonylurea use
Octreotide can be given to inhibit insulin release from the pancreas.

If there is suspected alcohol abuse or malnutrition
Give thiamine to avoid Wernicke's encephalopathy.

Monitor blood glucose closely and replace as needed
Start IVF of D_5 1/2 NS
Admit pts with
Profound hypoglycemia that requires frequent correction and monitoring
Hypoglycemia caused by sulfonylurea or long-acting insulin use
Suicidal ingestions
Lack of follow-up

Most pts will be able to be safely discharged home if
Their blood glucose remains normal post-correction.
Their mental status has returned to normal.
They tolerate an oral diet.
They are observed for a while in the ED.

IV
Pulmonary

Asthma Exacerbation

S **What are the pt's current symptoms?**
Common symptoms include:
- Cough
- Chest tightness
- Dyspnea
- Wheezing

Does the pt have a history of asthma?
If no prior history, consider an alternative diagnosis or reactive airway disease.
How often does the pt come to the ED for an exacerbation?
- Marker of how well controlled the asthma is.

Does the pt know what triggered this event?
Most asthmatics also suffer from allergies and know what triggered their attack. If no trigger is obvious, consider an infection.
Common triggers include:
- Fragrances
- Cold
- Smoke
- Animal dander
- Respiratory infections
- Exercise
- Drugs/Medications

Has the pt aspirated or choked on something? Exclude foreign-body aspiration.

Has the pt done any self-treatment or received any treatment before coming to the ED?
Will help direct your ED management and disposition.

Has the pt ever been intubated for an asthma exacerbation?
Correlates with the degree of asthma the pt has and may predict things to come.

What medications is the pt taking?
Ask specifically about all inhalers and if any new medications have been started recently.
When was the last time the pt was on oral steroids? Typically correlates with the last exacerbation.

Does the pt check peak flows at home or know the baseline?
Helps quantify the severity of the current asthma exacerbation.

What other medical problems does the pt have?
Congestive heart failure (CHF) exacerbations can present with dyspnea and wheezing and may be difficult to differentiate from an asthma or chronic obstructive pulmonary disease exacerbation.

Obtain a social history
Ask specifically about smoking or exposure to second-hand smoke.
Employment history may elicit exposure to chemicals or fumes.

O **Check pt's vital signs**
Perform a physical exam
General: Can the pt speak in full sentences? Is he or she in distress?
HEENT: Note any signs of a upper respiratory infection (URI) or cyanosis.
Lungs: Wheezing? Egophony? Signs of consolidation? What is the inspiration-to-expiration ratio?
- Is the pt using accessory muscles to breathe?
- May not hear wheezing in severe cases because of diminished air flow.

Cardiac: Tachycardia is common.
Neurologic: Mental status changes can be seen with hypoxia.

Check peak flows
Helps quantify the severity of the asthma exacerbation. It is better if baseline values are known.
Normal values depend on age and height. In general:
- 400–600 Normal
- 100–300 Moderate Exacerbation
- < 100 Severe Exacerbation

Check a CXR if
- New-onset asthma
- Altered level of consciousness
- Pneumonia or infection suspected
- Fever

Consider obtaining the following labs
ABG: Evaluates the degree of hypoxia, and elevated CO_2 may indicate impending respiratory failure.
CBC: WBCs may be elevated with infection.

A
Asthma Exacerbation -or-
Reactive Airway Disease
Differential Diagnosis
- Pneumonia
- Foreign body
- Bronchitis
- Allergic reaction
- Pneumothorax
- CHF

P
Maintain SpO_2 > 92%. Add supplemental oxygen as needed.
If pt is in extreme respiratory distress or showing signs of fatigue
Consider intubation or trial of continuous positive airway pressure (CPAP).

Start nebulizer treatments with albuterol (short-acting β-agonist) and/or ipratropium
Consider a continuous nebulizer treatment.
Metered-dose inhalers (MDIs) are equally efficacious to nebulizer in the nonacute setting, but pt's ability to use an MDI in the acute setting tends to be limited.

Administer oral or IV steroids.
Mainstay of therapy and helps relieve airway inflammation.

Consider administering magnesium sulfate.
Effective bronchial dilator, especially in children, where it has been shown to decrease the need for intubation.

Consider starting Heliox (helium-oxygen mixture)
Helium decreases airflow resistance and has been shown to decrease the need for intubation.
May need to be combined with CPAP to ensure that nebulizer medications enter the airways and do not settle in the mouth.

Discharge pts with mild exacerbations who have improved while in the ED
Most pts should be discharged with a 5-day course of oral steroids.
Ensure close follow-up with their primary care provider.

Admit pts who exhibited or who required
- Mental status changes
- Hypoxia
- Required Heliox
- Concurrent pneumonia
- Required CPAP, intubation

S | What are the pt's current symptoms?
Common symptoms include:
- Dyspnea
- Productive cough
- Decreased exercise tolerance
- Weakness
- Easy fatigability
- Chest tightness

Does the pt know what triggered this event?
Common triggers are:
- Noncompliance with medications
- Upper respiratory infection/Infections
- Fragrances/Odors
- Pet dander

Does the pt smoke?
Smoking causes approximately 80% to 90% of chronic obstructive pulmonary disease (COPD) cases. Only 20% are caused by occupational exposure or $\alpha 1$-antitrypsin deficiency (a rare disorder that can cause emphysema).

What medical problems does the pt have?
Congestive heart failure (CHF) and COPD are commonly present in the same person, and differentiating an exacerbation between the two can be difficult.

What medications is the pt currently taking?
Ask about recent antibiotic usage.
Have any medications been changed recently?

Obtain a social history
Environmental and occupational exposure may cause exacerbations.
Document tobacco history.

O | Evaluate pt's vital signs
Note respiration rate and SpO_2.

Perform a physical exam
General: Note the degree of respiratory distress and accessory muscle use.
- Can the pt speak in a full sentence?

Lungs: Wheezing? Diminished air movement? Egophony?
Cardiac: Increased jugular venous distention? Tachycardia? Murmurs? Exclude CHF from diagnosis.
Extremities: Clubbing? Cyanosis? Edema?
Neurologic: Mental status change with hypoxia?

Check a CXR
May see hyperinflation as evidenced by flattened diaphragms, hyperlucency, and bullae.
Exclude pneumonia, pneumothorax, and pulmonary edema.

Consider B-type natriuretic peptide (BNP) if alternative diagnosis of CHF is possible
BNP level < 100 essentially excludes CHF exacerbation.
BNP can be elevated in the 100–300 range with cor pulmonale and right ventricle strain seen in end-stage COPD.

Consider the following labs
CBC: May have elevated WBC as a result of infection or distress of hypoxia. Exclude anemia.

ABG: Evaluate degree of oxygenation and ventilatory status. Most chronic COPD pts have a baseline respiratory acidosis (elevated CO_2) that is well compensated. Arterial pH < 7.3 signifies an acute deterioration.

Consider ECG, cardiac enzymes
Exclude coronary ischemia. ECG typically shows right ventricle (RV) strain, RV hypertrophy, and low QRS voltage.

A COPD Exacerbation
COPD is the fourth leading cause of death and claims the lives of approximately 110,000 Americans annually.

Differential Diagnosis
- CHF exacerbation
- Asthma exacerbation
- Pneumonia
- Acute bronchitis

P Provide supplemental oxygen
Maintain SpO_2 > 92% or PaO_2 > 60.
If respiratory effort significantly decreases with oxygen therapy, consider intubation.

Consider trial of continuous positive airway pressure or intubation
If severe respiratory distress with or without hypoxia

Administer inhaled bronchodilators
β-agonist (albuterol) and anticholinergics (ipratropium) are the mainstay of therapy.

Start an antibiotic. Latest guidelines and research support that antibiotics decrease the duration and severity of a COPD exacerbation.

Start systemic steroids
IV or oral steroids are equally efficacious if the pt is able to take oral meds.
Play less of a role in emphysema, although most COPD pts also have a component of bronchospasm and bronchial inflammation.

Strongly encourage smoking cessation
Studies show that a single 5-minute conversation with a physician will significantly increase the pt's chance of quitting.

Discharge pts who have mild symptoms, have responded in the ED, and have close follow-up
Discharge meds should include:
- Oral steroids for a 5- to 7-day course
- Inhaled bronchodilators
- Oral antibiotic
- Consider inhaled steroid

Admit all pts with moderate to severe symptoms

Pleural Effusion — Pulmonary

S

What are the pt's current symptoms?
Most pts will be asymptomatic, and the pleural effusion will be an incidental finding on CXR or CT scan.
May experience:
- Pleuritic chest pain
- Shortness of breath
- Cough
- Fever

Has the pt been involved in a recent trauma?
Need to exclude hemothorax or bloody effusion, which has a higher risk of becoming an empyema.

Does the pt have any risk factors for a pleural effusion?
Transudative effusions are seen with:
- Congestive heart failure (CHF)
- Pulmonary embolism
- Nephrotic syndrome
- Severe hypothyroidism
- Cirrhosis

Exudative effusions are seen with:
- Pneumonia
- Cancer
- Pericarditis
- Pancreatitis
- Esophageal rupture
- Empyema
- Trauma
- Chylothorax

Does the pt have any other medical problems?
May help elicit a possible cause for the effusion.

Is the pt taking any medications?
Amiodarone use has been linked to pleural effusions.

O

Assess pt's vital signs
Note fever and SpO_2.

Perform a physical exam
General: Is the pt in any distress?
HEENT: Note any jugular venous distension.
Lungs: May have decreased breath sounds in the bases, dullness to percussion, or decreased tactile fremitus. Note any wheezing or bronchial breath sounds.
Cardiac: In severe cases, heart sounds may be muffled and point of maximum impulse displaced. Note any murmurs, S3 and/or S4 as evidence of CHF.
Abdomen: Note any masses, distention, ascites, or tenderness.
Extremities: Pedal edema?

Obtain a CXR
Will show blunting of the costophrenic angle and an air-fluid level.
Lateral decubitus films can help differentiate effusion from pulmonary consolidation.
- Fluid will layer out.

Loculated pleural effusions may be difficult to see on CXR.

Consider chest CT scan
Highly sensitive for pleural effusions and will show loculations.
Can evaluate surrounding structure and may elicit a cause for the effusion.

Consider a diagnostic thoracentesis
If etiology is unknown or pt is having severe respiratory distress
Localize area of maximum dullness. Ultrasound can help localize the largest fluid collection.
Thoracentesis needle is inserted perpendicular to the skin over the rib at the area of the greatest fluid collection.

Aspirate fluid and send for:
- Glucose
- Lactate dehydrogenase (LDH)
- Rheumatoid serologies
- Amylase
- Protein
- pH
- Cell count
- Gram stain
- Cytology

Analyze fluid. Fluid is an exudate if:
- Fluid LDH: Serum LDH > 0.6
- Fluid protein: Serum protein > 0.5
- Fluid LDH > two-thirds the upper limit of LDH in serum

Obtain a post-procedure CXR to rule out iatrogenic pneumothorax.

Obtain the following labs
CBC: May see leukocytosis.
LFT, amylase, lipase: Rule out liver disease or pancreatitis.

A **Pleural Effusion**
Normal pleural fluid is < 15 mL and acts as a lubricant between the parietal and visceral pleura.
Most common causes are cancer, CHF, pneumonia, and pulmonary embolus.
Exudative effusions are caused by inflammation of the pleura or disruption of lymphatic flow, resulting in fluid accumulation.
Transudative effusions are caused by increased hydrostatic pressures, resulting in capillary leak.
See risk factors for possible causes.

P **Most effusions are asymptomatic and require no special treatment**
Treat the underlying disorder, and the pleural effusion should resolve on its own.

Thoracentesis should be performed to diagnose cause or relieve respiratory distress
Administer supplemental oxygen to maintain SpO$_2$ > 92%
Consider chest tube placement for
Hemothorax
Empyema
Large complicated parapneumonic effusions that may result in empyema

Admission determination should be based on degree of symptoms and underlying disorder
Pts with moderate to large pleural effusion with no known cause should be admitted for further evaluation.

S | What are the pt's current symptoms?
Common symptoms include:
- Cough
- Fever
- Pleuritic chest pain
- Dyspnea
- Nausea/vomiting
- Wheezing
- Generalized fatigue
- Rigors
- Hemoptysis
- Mental status changes may be the only symptom in the elderly.

Obtain a past medical history
Comorbid illnesses can increase the severity of infection.
- Diabetes
- Chronic obstructive pulmonary disease (COPD)
- Cystic fibrosis
- Cancer
- Asthma

Does the pt live in a nursing home or recently been hospitalized?
Increases the risk of nosocomial pneumonia and changes the choice of empiric antibiotics.

Is there a history of alcohol abuse or loss of consciousness?
Increases risk for aspiration pneumonia.

Does the pt have any risk factors for tuberculosis (TB)?
These include living in or originating from a developing country, age (< 5 yrs, middle-aged and elderly men), alcoholism and/or drug addiction, HIV, diabetes, lodging house dwellers, immunosuppression, close contact with TB-positive pts, previous gastrectomy, and smoking.
If TB is suspected, immediately place the pt in isolation.

Does the pt have a history of recurrent pneumonias?
Increases suspicion for aspiration or postobstructive pneumonia.

Has the pt been on antibiotics recently?
Will affect your choice of empiric antibiotics and disposition.

Has the pt been vaccinated for *Streptococcus pneumonia* or *Haemophilus influenzae*?
Reduces risk and severity of illness but does not afford 100% immunity.

Obtain a social history
Determine any alcohol or tobacco history.
Have there been any occupational exposure, suggestive of hypersensitivity pneumonitis?

O | Assess pt's vital signs
Note fever and SpO_2.

Perform a physical exam
General: Is the pt in distress? Diaphoresis?
Lungs: Wheezing? Egophony? Decreased breath sounds? Tactile fremitus? Increased work of breathing?
Cardiac: Tachycardia?
Extremities: Cyanosis?
Neurologic: Mental status changes?

Obtain a CXR
Look for air bronchograms, infiltrate, effusion, and/or opacification.
Lower lobe findings typically present with more severe hypoxia.

Check the following labs
CBC: Leukocytosis?
Sputum culture: Rarely helpful but recommended.
Blood cultures × 2: If pt is going to be hospitalized, although < 10% isolate the causative agent.
Legionella urine antigen: If suspicion and incidence in your area support ordering.

A ### Pneumonia
Community-acquired pneumonia (CAP): Common pathogens include *Streptococcus pneumonia, Haemophilus influenzae, Mycoplasma pneumoniae, Legionella, Moraxella catarrhalis*, and viruses.
Nosocomial pneumonia: Common organisms are *Staphylococcus aureus, Pseudomonas aeruginosa*, and CAP organisms.
Aspiration pneumonia: Above organisms in addition to anaerobic.

-or-

Tuberculosis   -or-
Acute Bronchitis
Typically has the same presentation as pneumonia with a normal CXR.

Differential Diagnosis
- Hypersensitivity pneumonitis
- Asthma
- Congestive heart failure
- Foreign-body aspiration
- COPD
- Bronchitis

P ### Administer supplemental oxygen to maintain SpO$_2$ > 92%
If hypoxia is severe and not responding to supplemental oxygen, intubate.

If TB is suspected, isolate pt
Start antibiotics
CAP: If being discharged home, consider fluoroquinolone or macrolide.
- If being hospitalized, third- or fourth-generation cephalosporin and macrolide.

Nosocomial: Admit pt and start anti-*Pseudomonas* cephalosporin/penicillin and gentamicin or fluoroquinolone. Consider adding vancomycin if pt has history of methicillin-resistant *Staphylococcus aureus*.
Aspiration: Fluoroquinolone plus clindamycin/metronidazole
Bronchitis: Fluoroquinolone or macrolide

If HIV-positive, start antibiotic coverage for *Pneumocystis carinii*
Pts who are well appearing, well oxygenated, and have no comorbid conditions may be discharged
Admit all pts with hypoxemia, hemodynamic instability, mental status changes, or toxic appearance
Pts who have failed outpatient therapy should also be admitted.

S — What are the pt's symptoms?
Typical symptoms include:
- Sudden onset of pleuritic chest pain on the affected side
- Dyspnea   - Tachypnea   - Cough

Does the pt have any risk factors for a pneumothorax?
- Smoking   - Trauma   - Atmospheric pressure change
- Genetic predisposition (e.g., α1-antitrypsin deficiency, Marfan syndrome)
- Increased incidence in young, thin, tall men.

Has the pt been involved in any trauma?
Penetrating trauma has the highest risk for pneumothorax.

Is there a prior history of pneumothorax?
Recurrent pneumothoraxes may need surgical intervention to prevent future occurrences.

Does the pt have any medical conditions?
Any disease that can affect pulmonary reserve (e.g., chronic obstructive pulmonary disease [COPD], cancer, cystic fibrosis, pulmonary embolus) will make the signs and symptoms of a pneumothorax more severe.

Obtain a social history
Smoking and cocaine inhalation have been associated with pneumothorax.

Perform a review of symptoms
May elicit symptoms consistent with an alternative diagnosis (e.g., pulmonary embolus, pneumonia, bronchitis).

O — Check pt's vital signs
Ensure that pt is hemodynamically stable.
- Hypotension, tachycardia, and tachypnea are seen with tension pneumothorax. Check SpO_2.

Perform a physical exam
General: Is there any respiratory distress?
HEENT: Is there jugular venous distention or tracheal deviation? These are signs of tension pneumothorax.
Lungs: Are breath sounds equal bilaterally? Typically will have diminished breath sounds on the affected side.
Chest: Any signs of trauma? Look for penetrating wounds.
Cardiac: Are the heart sounds displaced or muffled? Can occur with tension pneumothorax.
Extremities: Any signs of cyanosis?

If there are signs of tension pneumothorax, immediately proceed with needle decompression
Do NOT confirm suspicion with a CXR.

Obtain a CXR
Absence of vascular lung marking peripheral to a **radiolucent line** is diagnostic of a pneumothorax.

Upright expiratory CXR maximizes visualization.

> CXR may miss an anterior pneumothorax.
> - A lateral decubitus CXR may aid in the visualization.

Consider chest CT scan
Highly sensitive and will detect a pneumothorax missed on CXR.

No laboratory studies are needed, although ABG may show hypoxemia and respiratory alkalosis

A Pneumothorax
Free air in the pleural space
Four types:
- Primary: No underlying medical condition
- Secondary: Associated with an underlying lung disorder (e.g., COPD)
- Traumatic: Caused by a trauma
- Iatrogenic: Result of a medical procedure (e.g., central line)

Tension Pneumothorax
A TRUE MEDICAL EMERGENCY
Occurs when air continues to leak from the lung into the pleural space and is unable to escape, increasing intrathoracic pressure. As the pressure increases, venous blood return is impaired and eventually stopped, leading to cardiac arrest.

Differential Diagnosis
- Pneumonia
- Pulmonary embolus
- Rib fracture
- Chest wall contusion
- COPD exacerbation
- Asthma exacerbation
- Pleuritis
- Myocardial infarction

P Tension Pneumothorax
Immediate needle decompression is needed. Insert a 14-gauge needle in the second intercostal space at the midclavicular line. Diagnosis is confirmed when a rush of air is heard on placement and there is immediate improvement in blood pressure and respiratory effort.
Definitive treatment with tube thoracotomy is needed because needle decompression is a temporizing measure.

Pneumothorax
Small primary pneumothoraxes (< 15%) in a hemodynamically stable pt can be observed in the ED for 6 hrs. If no change is seen on follow-up CXR, pt can be discharged home with close follow-up.
Pts with a > 15% pneumothorax, co-morbid conditions, hemodynamic instability, or poor pulmonary reserve should have a pigtail catheter or tube thoracotomy placed.
Traumatic pneumothoraxes should be treated with the placement of a pigtail catheter or tube thoracotomy. A pigtail catheter is better tolerated, but is not large enough in caliber to evacuate blood, and should be restricted to pure pneumothoraxes.

Pulmonary Edema

S **What are the pt's current symptoms?**
Typical symptoms include:
- Dyspnea
- Anxiety
- Tachypnea
- Orthopnea
- Diaphoresis
- Weakness

Determine the type of onset and duration of the pt's symptoms?
Abrupt onset is seen with myocardial infarction, acute mitral regurgitation, hypertensive urgency, or toxic exposure.
Gradual onset is consistent with congestive heart failure (CHF) exacerbation or chronic toxic exposure.

Has the pt been involved in a recent trauma?
Pulmonary edema has been reported with central nervous system (CNS) injuries, trauma, seizures, aspiration, and with reexpansion of the lung after treatment for pneumothorax or hemothorax.

Does the pt have any other medical problems?
Common associated diseases include:
- Aortic stenosis
- Renal failure
- Hyperthyroidism
- Mitral regurgitation
- Liver failure
- Seizures
- CHF
- Hypertension
- CNS injury

Obtain a social history to include occupational exposures
Chemical exposure and inhalation injuries can cause pulmonary edema.
Opioids and cocaine inhalation have been associated with pulmonary edema.

What medication does the pt take?
Will help determine risk factors and medical problems if the pt is unable to communicate.

O **Evaluate the pt's vital signs**
Note SpO_2, respiratory rate, and blood pressure.

Perform a physical exam
General: Respiratory distress? Able to speak in full sentences? (Inability to complete a full sentence correlates with degree of respiratory distress.) Any signs of trauma?
HEENT: Jugular venous distention elevated? Any soot or burns around the nose and mouth? (seen with inhalation injuries)
Lungs: Rales? Wheezing? Decreased breath sounds? Accessory muscle use?
Cardiac: Tachycardia? Murmurs? Gallop? Seen with CHF.
Abdomen: Ascites? Seen with CHF.
Extremities: Pedal edema, diminished pulses.

Obtain a CXR
Increased vascular markings (cephalization), pleural effusion, alveolar infiltrates, cardiomyopathy, and Kerley B Lines (short linear markings in the lung periphery) may all be seen with pulmonary edema.

Obtain an ECG
Exclude myocardial infarction and myocardial ischemia.

Consider obtaining the following labs
CBC to exclude anemia and secondary high-output cardiac failure as cause
BUN, creatinine to evaluate renal function.

LFT to exclude liver failure.
Cardiac enzymes to exclude myocardial infarction.
BNP to exclude CHF.

A **Pulmonary Edema**
The leakage of intravascular fluid into the pulmonary interstitium and air spaces.
Causes divided into two categories.
- *Cardiogenic*: Includes valvular heart disease, cardiomyopathy, pericarditis, myocardial infarction, hypertensive crisis, and volume overload. The pulmonary edema is caused by increased hydrostatic pressure in the pulmonary capillaries, causing intravascular fluid to leak out.
- *Noncardiogenic*: Includes lung reexpansion, occupational or inhalation injuries, drugs (e.g., opioids, cocaine), aspiration, trauma, CNS injury, or sepsis. The pulmonary edema is caused by damage to the pulmonary capillary permeability, which allows fluid to leak out of the intravascular space.

Differential Diagnosis
- Chronic obstructive pulmonary disease
- Adult respiratory distress syndrome
- Pneumonia
- CHF

P **Provide supplemental oxygen**
Maintain SpO_2 > 92%.
Intubate or place on continuous positive airway pressure if in severe respiratory distress.

Cardiogenic Pulmonary Edema
Maximize cardiac function. Goals of therapy are to normalize afterload, preload, and cardiac output.
- If blood pressure is markedly elevated, give vasodilators to decrease afterload.
- Diurese pt with loop diuretics if volume overload is suspected.
- Treat myocardial ischemia and infarction if present. Emergent revascularization may be required.
- Consider inotropes (e.g., dopamine and/or dobutamine) for pump failure (inadequate cardiac output).

Most pts will require admission. All should be admitted to a monitored bed, and an ICU setting should be considered for any pt who requires mechanical ventilations or is hemodynamically unstable.
Pts with mild symptoms who improve with treatment in the ED, have normal vital signs and diagnostic tests, and have close follow-up can be considered for discharge.

Noncardiogenic Pulmonary Edema
Generally a self-limited process, and only supportive care is needed.
Treat causative agent and provide respiratory support.
All pts should be admitted and observed closely for progression of the edema.

S | What are the pt's current symptoms?
Common symptoms include:
- Pleuritic chest pain
- Dyspnea
- Cough
- Hemoptysis
- Syncope
- Diaphoresis
- Anxiety
- Restlessness

Does the pt have any risk factors for deep venous thrombosis (DVT)?
(See Venous Thrombosis p. 24.)

Does the pt have a history of DVT, pulmonary embolus (PE), or hypercoagulable state?
Greater risk for repeat occurrence

Does the pt have any medical problems?
Preexisting pulmonary disorders will decrease pulmonary reserve and increase symptoms.

Cancer, lupus, obesity, and pregnancy are associated with hypercoagulable states and increased PE risk.

Has the pt recently delivered a baby?
Amniotic fluid embolus can occur post-delivery.

Has the pt suffered any long-bone fractures?
Recent fracture is associated with fat embolus.

Is the pt taking any medication?
May be on warfarin from prior DVT/PE; or estrogen, which increases thrombus risk.
Helps elicit other medical disorders.

Obtain a social history
Smoking increases the risk of thrombus formation.
IV drug abusers can suffer a pulmonary embolus from injected foreign bodies.

O | Check pt's vital signs
Pay attention to SpO_2 and ensure that the pt is hemodynamically stable. Pts can present in cardiac arrest or shock.
May have a low-grade fever.

Perform a physical exam
General: Is the pt in respiratory distress?
Lungs: Wheezing? Rales? May hear diminished breath sounds or pleural rub over the affected area.
Cardiac: Tachycardia? Murmur? Right ventricular (RV) heave?
Extremities: Lower extremity swelling? Homans' sign? Calf tenderness?

Obtain CXR
Usually normal. May see a Hampton's hump (wedge-shaped infiltrate) or Westermark sign (area of decreased pulmonary vasculature). Pleural effusion may be present.

Obtain the following labs
ABG: May show hypoxemia and respiratory alkalosis.
PT, INR, PTT: Baseline studies before starting any anticoagulation medications.
D-dimer: A degradation product of fibrin, which is elevated in any state that causes a thrombus. Nonspecific but can help rule out the diagnosis in low-risk pts.
CBC: Baseline study
UA: Fat molecules in urine help secure diagnosis of fat embolus.
BUN, Creatinine: Exclude renal insufficiency if LMWH is to be used.

Obtain a diagnostic study
Individual test will depend on the availability or expertise of your individual institution.
Chest CT scan, helical spiral CT: Very sensitive for proximal PEs but can miss distal/peripheral PE.
Ventilation/perfusion scan: Sensitivity dependent on pretest probability. Underlying lung disease can affect the interpretation of the study.
Pulmonary angiogram: The gold standard, but the most invasive test and requires specially trained staff.

Two negative studies are required to exclude the diagnosis if your pretest probability is high.

Obtain an ECG
Most common finding is sinus tachycardia. May see RV strain as evidenced by the classic $S_1Q_3T_3$ pattern.

Consider lower-extremity Dopplers
Does not confirm the diagnosis, but if positive will increase the likelihood of PE and dictate the same treatment be started.

Consider echocardiogram
Look for evidence of RV strain and dysfunction, which is the criteria for giving thrombolytics.

A Pulmonary Embolus

Virchow's triad (i.e., venous stasis, hypercoagulable state, endothelial damage) describes the conditions that increase the risk for PE.

An embolus can be a thrombus, fat particles, or amniotic fluid.

Differential Diagnosis
- Congestive heart failure
- Myocardial infarction
- Pneumonia
- Pneumothorax
- Asthma
- Chronic obstructive pulmonary disease
- Pleurisy

P Provide supplemental oxygen. Maintain $SpO_2 > 92\%$.
Treat hypotension, if present, with IV fluids
Consider dobutamine if no response to IV fluids.

Start anticoagulation unless contraindicated
Unfractionated heparin versus LMWH [contraindicated in renal failure] at therapeutic doses.
Can start warfarin on day 1 if no invasive procedures are planned.

Consider inferior vena cava filter placement. Indicated for:
Pts with contraindications for anticoagulation
Recurrent PE despite adequate anticoagulation
Pts with tenuous cardiopulmonary status, where an additional PE can be life ending

Consider systemic thrombolytics
Indicated in cases where there is documented RV strain and dysfunction by echocardiogram.

Consider pulmonary embolectomy in cases of refractory shock
Admit all pts to a monitored bed or ICU depending on status

V
Gastrointestinal

Abdominal Aortic Aneurysm

S **What are the pt's current symptoms?**
Unruptured aneurysms are typically asymptomatic, although pts may experience vague abdominal or back pain.
Ruptured aneurysms typically present with:
- Severe abdominal or back pain
- Weakness/fatigue
- Nausea/Vomiting
- Syncope
- Lightheadedness

Does the pt have hematemesis?
- May signify an aortoenteric fistula. Normally associated with prior abdominal aortic aneurysm (AAA) repair.

Does the pt have a history of AAA?
Useful to know the last known size to make comparisons. Aneurysms typically grow 0.3 to 0.5 cm per year. Helpful to predict current size.

Does the pt have any risk factors for AAA?
- Atherosclerosis   - Hypertension   - Marfan syndrome
- Male gender   - Tobacco use   - Peripheral vascular disease
- Age > 60

Does the pt have any other medical problems?
Does the pt take any medications? Have any doses been missed?
Uncontrolled hypertension can exacerbate rupture of an aneurysm.
Ensure that pt is not on any anticoagulants.

Has the pt had any unexplained weight loss or early satiety?
Superior mesenteric artery syndrome is where the AAA compresses the duodenum, causing nausea, vomiting, and weight loss.

O **Evaluate the pt's vital signs**
Hypertension will exacerbate ruptures, and hypotension may be seen with severe bleeding.

Perform a physical exam
Abdomen: Rigidity? Guarding? Listen for abdominal bruit. May be able to feel a pulsatile mass. Do not palpate too hard because it may cause rupture.

Skin: Look for signs of retroperitoneal hematoma. Grey-Turner's sign is ecchymosis and hemorrhage along the flank. Cullen's sign is ecchymosis over the periumbilical region.

Neurologic: May have weakness or numbness in the lower extremities.

Obtain the following labs
CBC: May show anemia but is likely to be normal acutely. Establishes baseline.
PT, INR, PTT: Rule out coagulopathy.
Electrolytes, BUN, creatinine: Ensure normal renal function because aneurysm can involve renal arteries and cause renal failure.
Type and cross: Ensure that blood is available in case the pt requires it.

Obtain a diagnostic study
Abdominal Ultrasound: Easy bedside test available in most teaching EDs. Can make the diagnosis of aneurysm but insensitive for rupture.

Abdominal CT scan: Highly sensitive for aneurysm and rupture, although can only be done on stable pts. May help establish an alternative diagnosis.

Plain x-rays: Insensitive, but 55% to 85% of AAAs can be seen on plain films. Classic findings are dilated calcified aortic wall, loss of psoas or renal shadow, or paravertebral soft tissue mass.

A Abdominal Aortic Aneurysm

Most AAAs originate below the renal arteries, and rupture may cause obstruction of renal, mesenteric, or spinal arteries with secondary renal failure, abdominal pain caused by bowel ischemia, and lower extremity paralysis, respectively.

The normal aorta is < 2 cm in diameter, and the likelihood of rupture increases with aneurysms > 5 cm. Asymptomatic aneurysms > 5 cm should be repaired electively.

Differential Diagnosis
- Renal colic
- Mesenteric schemia
- Diverticulitis
- Myocardial infarction
- Aortic dissection
- Peptic ulcer disease

P If asymptomatic
Elective repair if AAA > 5 cm

- 5% perioperative mortality with elective surgery.

Serial exams and management of hypertension, atherosclerosis if AAA < 5 cm
Discharge pt if AAA is incidental finding, < 5 cm, and pt has close follow-up.

If symptomatic
Hypotension: Treat by administering packed red blood cells and IV fluids.
If bedside ultrasound shows AAA and pt is unstable, pt should proceed to surgery without any additional diagnostic studies.

- Approximately 50% perioperative mortality with emergent repair following rupture.

If hemodynamically stable, pt may undergo additional testing to rule out alternative diagnosis and evaluate extent of involvement of associated vascular structures.
Admit all pts.
- Most will require ICU admission because they can deteriorate quickly.

Appendicitis

S **Does the pt have any abdominal pain? Where is it located?**
Classic abdominal pain starts in the epigastric/periumbilical area and migrates to the right lower quadrant (RLQ) (McBurney's point).
Pts at the extremes of age are more likely to have an atypical presentation.
- Pediatric pts may only present with lethargy.
- Elderly pts may present with mental status changes or vague symptoms.

Does the pain radiate anywhere?
Depending on location of the appendix, pain may radiate to the groin or flank.

Does anything exacerbate the pain?
Peritoneal pain is typically worsened by walking, hopping, or hitting bumps on the car ride to the hospital.

Does the pt have any associated symptoms?
- Anorexia   - Nausea/Vomiting   - Fever

Is the pt pregnant?
The pain in pregnancy can be anywhere in the abdomen, and the pt may have an atypical presentation.

When was the pt's last menses?
Ensure that pt is not pregnant and at risk for an ectopic pregnancy.

Does the pt have any other medical problems?
May help elicit an alternative diagnosis (e.g., diverticulitis).

Has the pt been on antibiotics recently?
Pt is more likely to present with an atypical presentation or prolonged mild symptoms.

O **Evaluate pt's vital signs**
Is there a low-grade fever? Is pt hemodynamically stable?

Perform a physical exam
General: Does the pt appear toxic?
Abdomen: Point tenderness? Rebound? Guarding? Any pain with heel tap or pelvic shake?
- *Psoas sign:* Increased RLQ pain with extension of the right hip.
- *Obturator sign:* Increased RLQ pain with extension and internal rotation of right hip.
- *Rovsing's sign:* RLQ pain with palpation of the left lower quadrant.

Gyn: Adnexal mass or tenderness? Vaginal bleeding? Cervical motion tenderness (CMT)?
- Rule out alternative diagnosis.
- CMT can be seen with any disease process that causes peritoneal signs.

GU: Any testicular masses or tenderness? Penile discharge?
Rectal: Check hemocult. Rectal pain or tenderness?

Obtain the following labs
CBC: May see a leukocytosis.
UA: Should be normal but may see hematuria and pyuria.
β-hCG: Exclude unknown pregnancy.

Obtain a diagnostic study
Abdominal Ultrasound: Can show dilation of the appendix and abscess. Helpful if positive, but if negative, will need to evaluate with a CT scan.
- Consider as a first-line test in very thin individuals or those where there is a suspicion of a pelvic pathology (e.g., ectopic pregnancy, ovarian cyst).

Abdominal CT Scan: With oral contrast can show > 90% of appendicitis. Classic findings include appendix wall thickening, periappediceal inflammation, and/or abscess.

- Very thin individuals make interpretation of CT extremely difficult because there is no separation between the loops of bowel.

A Appendicitis
Peak incidence between ages 10 to 30. Results when the appendical lumen is obstructed.

Differential Diagnosis
- Pancreatitis
- Ectopic pregnancy
- Nephrolithiasis
- Diverticulitis
- Pelvic inflammatory disease
- Gastroenteritis
- Ovarian cyst
- Testicular torsion
- Intestinal obstruction

P Start IV fluids
Administer appropriate pain medication
Narcotics have not been shown to mask the signs of appendicitis and may even help make the diagnosis because they can help eliminate guarding and anxiety that confound the exam.

Start antibiotics
3rd-generation cephalosporin or penicillin/β-lactamase inhibitor
Add anaerobic coverage with clindamycin or metronidazole if perforation is suspected.

Consult a general surgeon
If pt is male and has classic findings, a surgeon may proceed to surgery without a diagnostic study. Appendectomy is treatment of choice.
Admit pt for serial abdominal exams if diagnosis is not absolute after exam and diagnostic studies are complete.

Consider discharge
If pt has no peritoneal signs, is able to tolerate food and liquids, and has close follow-up
Pts should be observed in the ED for several hours and undergo serial abdominal exams to ensure that symptoms and exam do not worsen before discharging home.
Pts should not be discharged on antibiotics.

S | Does the pt have any abdominal pain?
Pain may be intermittent and colicky in nature or constant and crampy.
Pain is generally diffuse and difficult to localize.

Does the pt have nausea or vomiting?
May have bilious or fecal vomiting.

Does the pt have a history of abdominal surgery?
Any abdominal surgery increases the risk of adhesion formation and secondary bowel obstruction.
Recent surgery can be associated with an ileus and obstructive symptoms.

Does the pt have any hernias?
Incarceration of intestine within the hernia can cause strangulation.

When was the pt's last bowel movement?
Constipation and lack of flatus are signs of a complete obstruction. A pt may still pass flatus with a partial obstruction.

Does the pt have any other medical problems?
Cancer increases the risk of peritoneal metastasis and adhesion formation.
Ulcerative colitis and Crohn's disease can cause bowel inflammation and edema with secondary obstruction.

Is the pt taking any medications?
Obstruction is associated with opiates and anticholinergic medications.

Obtain a social history
Mesenteric ischemia is associated with tobacco use and peripheral vascular disease.

Obtain a review of symptoms
May help elicit an inciting cause of the obstruction.

O | Evaluate pt's vital signs
Fever may signify perforation and secondary infection.

Perform a physical exam
General: Is the pt toxic?
Abdomen: Distention? Tenderness? Hyperactive bowel sounds? Seen with obstruction. Rebound tenderness? Suspect perforation.
Rectal: Hemocult positive? Seen with peptic ulcer disease (PUD), ischemic bowel. Rectal tenderness? Suggests abscess or infection.

Obtain the following labs
CBC: May show leukocytosis.
Electrolytes, BUN, Creatinine: Exclude electrolyte disturbance or renal failure.
Lactic acid: Pain out of proportion to exam suggests mesenteric ischemia, which will have an elevated lactic acid level.

Obtain abdominal x-rays
Classic findings include:
- Dilated loops of bowel
    - Can localize obstruction by appearance of bowel. Colon has haustra that appear as lines that only partially cross the lumen of the colon. Small bowel has plicae circularis that completely cross the lumen.

- Air-fluid levels
- Lack of air in the rectum and distal bowel

Obtain a decubitus film to demonstrate free air if perforation is suspected.

Consider an abdominal CT scan
Can demonstrate obstruction and lead point (area where obstruction occurred). May show an alternative diagnosis.
Helps guide operative repair if needed.

A Bowel Obstruction
Etiologies include hernia with incarceration, volvulus, intussusception, fecal impaction, adhesions, foreign bodies, bowel ischemia, malignancy, or obstruction caused by medications or electrolyte disturbances.

Differential Diagnosis
- Gastroenteritis
- PUD
- Appendicitis
- Pancreatitis
- Diverticulitis
- Mesenteric ischemia
- Fecal impaction
- Pelvic inflammatory disease

P Start IV fluids. Keep pts NPO
Large fluid deficits may be present as a result of prolonged vomiting or third spacing.

Administer antiemetics for nausea
If nausea is persistent and there is a large amount of abdominal distention, consider placing a nasogastric tube to decompress the stomach.

Consider antibiotics
If perforation is suspected or if there is a possibility of infection as evidenced by elevated WBC or fever
Penicillin/β-lactamase inhibitor or 3rd-generation cephalosporin plus anaerobic coverage with metronidazole or clindamycin

Consult a general surgeon
If mesenteric ischemia, complete bowel obstruction, or strangulated hernia is suspected

Pts with partial obstruction or ileus can be admitted and observed
Treat causative illness if known (e.g., infection, electrolyte disturbance).

In children, colonic intussusception can be diagnosed and treated with a barium or air enema

Biliary Disease

S **Does the pt have risk factors for cholecystitis?**
- Obese (fat)
- Pregnant (fertile)
- Forty (years old)
- Female
- Recent weight loss
- History of gallstones

Does the pt have any pain?
Classic pain is in the right upper quadrant (RUQ) and exacerbated by eating meals with high fat content.
May radiate to the right shoulder.

How long has the pt been having symptoms?
Most pts will complain of intermittent RUQ pain after meals for several weeks or months before they present to the ED with severe pain.

Are there any associated symptoms?
Nausea and vomiting are common.

Does the pt have a fever or chills?
May be seen with cholangitis and acute cholecystitis.

Does the pt have any other medical problems?
Inflammatory bowel disease, cirrhosis, and diabetes increase risk for cholecystitis. A history of pancreatitis may suggest prior gallstones.

Obtain a social history
Heavy alcohol use can cause cirrhosis and fatty liver mimicking cholecystitis.

O **Evaluate the pt's vital signs**
Perform a physical exam
HEENT: Scleral icterus or mucous icterus? Seen with hyperbilirubinemia.

Abdomen: RUQ tenderness? Murphy's sign (pt stops inhaling when the RUQ is being palpated)? Seen with cholecystitis.

Rectal: Should be normal. Positive hemocult or blood on exam suggests alternative diagnosis.

Obtain the following labs
CBC: May see leukocytosis.
LFT: Alkaline phosphatase and bilirubin elevated in choledocholithiasis and may be elevated in cholecystitis.
Amylase/Lipase: Elevated in pancreatitis.

Obtain a diagnostic study
RUQ ultrasound:
- May show gallbladder and ductile dilation, gallbladder wall thickening, and pericholecystic fluid.
- "Gold Standard": Visualization of gallbladder can be affected by colonic gas. Pts should be NPO for 12 hrs before study.

Abdominal CT scan:
- Helpful to rule out masses and other pathology. Does not visualize the gallbladder well.

Hepatobiliary nuclear scan (HIDA):
- Shows uptake of radioactive isotope in the gallbladder if there is no obstruction. Delayed filling or no filling is diagnostic of cholecystitis.

Biliary Disease

A

Acute Cholecystitis
Acute inflammation and obstruction of the gallbladder resulting in persistent (> 6 hrs) pain.

Cholelithiasis
Gallstones with no evidence of obstruction or inflammation

Choledocholithiasis
Obstruction of the common bile duct

Cholangitis
An obstruction and ascending infection of the common bile duct

Biliary Colic
Intermittent obstruction of the cystic or common bile ducts result in pain. Precursor for acute cholecystitis.

Differential Diagnosis
- Gallstone pancreatitis
- Abdominal aortic aneurysm
- Peptic ulcer disease
- Pancreatitis
- Appendicitis
- Pyelonephritis
- Renal colic
- Diverticulitis
- Hepatitis

P

Start IV fluids and keep pt NPO
Provide pain relief
NSAIDs are effective in treating biliary colic.
Narcotics may be needed for more severe pain.

Cholelithiasis requires no treatment but increases the risk for acute cholecystitis in the future
Biliary colic can be treated with IV hydration and pain control
Keep pt NPO until symptoms resolve.
Future symptoms may be prevented by avoiding high-fat meals.

Acute cholecystitis
Continue IV fluids, keep NPO, and treat pain.
Consult General Surgery for cholecystectomy.
- May be delayed for several days to allow inflammation to decrease and prevent operative complications.

Start antibiotics to prevent complications and perforation.

Cholangitis
Requires aggressive treatment to prevent sepsis and hemodynamic collapse.
Start IV fluids, keep NPO, and treat pain.
Start broad-spectrum antibiotics with anaerobic coverage.
Consult General Surgery ASAP.
Arrange for emergent biliary drainage.
- May require percutaneous cholecystostomy tube if pt is too unstable for surgery.

Diarrhea

S

When was the pt's last bowel movement? How many bowel movements per day is the pt having?
Helpful to quantify the amount and frequency of the diarrhea.

Have the pt describe the appearance of the diarrhea
Watery diarrhea is associated with viral disease (e.g., Norwalk) and noninvasive (toxin-mediated) disease (e.g., *S. aureus*, *Bacillus cereus*, and *Clostridium perfringens*).
Bloody diarrhea is associated with invasive disease that is typically seen with *Shigella* and *E. coli* O157:H7.

Does the pt ever have to get up in the middle of the night to have a bowel movement?
Functional diarrhea is not typically associated with nocturnal symptoms. Suggests an infectious etiology.

Has the pt traveled recently?
Suggestive of giardiasis and traveler's diarrhea

Has the pt been on antibiotics recently?
Increased risk for *Clostridium difficile*

Does the pt have any underlying psychiatric disorder?
Bulimia and anorexia are associated with factitious diarrhea.

Does the pt have any associated symptoms?
Common symptoms include:
- Nausea/Vomiting
- Crampy abdominal pain
- Dehydration

Are any other close contacts ill? Did they eat together?
Attempt to isolate the source of potential food poisoning.

Does the pt have any other medical problems?
Inflammatory bowel disease (e.g., Crohn's/ulcerative colitis) may present with diarrhea during an acute flare.
Irritable bowel syndrome can be associated with diarrhea or constipation.

O

Evaluate the pt's vital signs
Check for a fever.
Tachycardia and hypotension seen with dehydration

Perform a physical exam
HEENT: Evaluate the mucous membranes and jugular venous distention for signs of dehydration.
Abdomen: Tenderness? Hypo-/hyperactive bowel sounds? Distention?
Rectal: Gross blood or hemocult positive? Rectal tenderness?

Consider obtaining the following labs
CBC: May see leukocytosis with invasive disease.
Stool for fecal fat and leukocytes: Fecal fat is seen with malabsorption syndromes.
   Leukocytes are seen with intestinal inflammation or invasive disease.
Stool for ova and parasites: May see *Giardia* or *Cryptosporidium*.

C. difficile toxin: Obtain in postantibiotic diarrhea to make diagnosis.
Stool culture: May isolate the causative agent.

A
Infectious Diarrhea - or-
Factitious Diarrhea
Self-induced diarrhea by laxative abuse or factitious reporting
-or-
Functional Diarrhea
Associated with irritable bowel disease and psychiatric disorders. Diarrhea cannot be shown to be caused by any structural or chemical abnormality.

Differential Diagnosis
- Malabsorption syndrome - Ischemic bowel
- Hyperthyroidism - HIV

P
Provide supportive care
Rehydrate the pt if there are signs of dehydration
Attempt oral hydration.
- The World Health Organization (WHO) has proven that oral hydration can be successful in repleting pts with significant diarrhea.

If needed, start IV fluids (e.g., NSS or lactated Ringer's).

Start an antidiarrheal agent
Bismuth subsalicylate: Reduces secretions, binds bacterial toxins, and possesses antimicrobial effects.
Loperamide: Inhibits peristalsis.
Atropine/diphenoxylate: Inhibits peristalsis.

Consider starting an antibiotic
Generally reserved for severe or invasive cases because it may prolong the carrier state.
Trimethoprim-sulfamethoxazole or a fluoroquinolone are generally recommended for empiric treatment because they have been shown to shorten the duration of diarrhea.
Metronidazole recommended for empiric treatment of suspected *Giardia* or *C. difficile*.
Oral vancomycin is drug of choice for *C. difficile*, although its use has been limited recently because of fears of inducing vancomycin-resistant enterococcus.

Admit any pt with hemodynamic instability or inability to tolerate oral liquids/food
Most pts can be discharged home after treatment in the ED

S **Does the pt have any abdominal pain?**
Commonly complains of left lower quadrant abdominal pain with diverticulitis, although may have pain anywhere.
Typical pain is nonradiating and may be increased by movement, although not positional.
Diverticulosis tends to be asymptomatic.

Has the pt had any fevers or chills?
Associated with diverticulitis

Does the pt have any associated symptoms?
Common symptoms include:
- Nausea/Vomiting   - Diarrhea/Constipation   - Anorexia

Has the pt experienced any rectal bleeding?
Painless rectal bleeding is the hallmark of diverticular bleeds; a common cause of lower GI bleeding in the elderly.

Does pt have a history of diverticulosis or diverticulitis?
Increased risk for diverticulitis in the future

Is the pt pregnant?
May see similar symptoms with an ectopic pregnancy.

Does the pt have any other medical problems?
History of peripheral vascular disease may suggest alternative diagnosis of mesenteric ischemia, and increases sensitivity to anemia with blood loss.
Pts with diabetes tend to have a higher rate of complications.

Obtain a review of symptoms
Vaginal discharge may suggest pelvic inflammatory disease (PID).
Dysuria, polyuria, or hematuria can be seen with urinary tract infection (UTI), pyelonephritis.

O **Evaluate the pt's vital signs**
Is the pt febrile?
Is the pt hemodynamically stable?

Perform a physical exam
Abdomen: Tenderness, rebound tenderness, and distention may be seen.
Rectal: Gross blood hemocult positive? May be seen with diverticular bleed. Rectal pain? Suggests colitis or abscess.

Obtain the following labs
CBC: Evaluate for leukocytosis and anemia.
β-hCG: Rule out pregnancy.
UA: Exclude UTI or pyelonephritis.
Type and cross if actively bleeding.

Consider a diagnostic study
Abdominal plain x-rays: Generally not helpful, although may demonstrate free air or signs of obstruction with air-fluid levels.
Abdominal CT scan: In diverticulitis, it will typically show diverticuli, pericolonic inflammation, and bowel wall thickening. May see abscess formation, perforation, or an alternative diagnosis.

- Should be obtained with oral contrast. IV contrast is not needed but will enhance the pericolonic inflammation.

Barium enema: Will show diverticuli but is contraindicated because of the risk of colonic overdistention and perforation.

Sigmoidoscopy/Colonoscopy: Can be obtained acutely for lower GI bleeding, but are contraindicated in the acute setting for diverticulitis for the same reasons as noted above.

A

Diverticulosis
Asymptomatic herniation of the colonic mucosa into the muscularis layer. Incidence is increased in the elderly and in societies that eat a low-fiber diet.

Diverticulitis
Acute inflammation and microabscess of one or more diverticulum, usually caused by an obstruction of the opening. Approximately 50% of pts with diverticulosis will develop diverticulitis over their lifetime.

Diverticular Bleed
Acute hemorrhage of a diverticulum. More common in the left colon.

Differential Diagnosis
- Appendicitis
- PID
- Inflammatory bowel disease
- Gastroenteritis
- Ectopic pregnancy
- Ischemic colitis
- UTI/Pyelonephritis

P

Initiate IV fluids and keep pt NPO

Diverticulosis
No treatment is needed. Typically an incidental finding found on CT scan or colonoscopy.

Diverticulitis
Start antibiotics. One possible combination is a fluoroquinolone and either clindamycin or metronidazole.

Treat pain with narcotics.

If pt's symptoms are mild, and there is no evidence of systemic disease, pt can be discharged home on oral antibiotics.

All pts with severe disease or inability to take oral medications need to be admitted for IV antibiotics and IV hydration.

Diverticular Bleed
Rule out upper GI bleed by placing NG tube and performing a gastric lavage.

Admit all pts. Pts who are hemodynamically unstable or at high risk for hemodynamic decompensation should be admitted to the ICU.

Transfuse blood as needed.

Consult Gastroenterology or a general surgeon so that a diagnostic procedure can be performed to localize the source of bleeding.

Foreign-Body Ingestion

S — What did the pt ingest?

> Small button batteries are the most worrisome because they require emergent removal if they become lodged in the esophagus. The battery can cause an alkaline burn and erode through the esophagus in as little as 4 hrs.

Does the pt have any difficulty breathing?
Object may cause airway obstruction or press on the trachea, obstructing air flow.

Can the pt swallow?
Obstruction in the esophagus can cause odynophagia or dysphagia.

Does the pt have any chest pain?
May be seen with esophageal perforation or after retching.

Does the pt have any symptoms?
Common symptoms include:
- Coughing/gagging
- Anxiety
- Nausea/Vomiting
- Hoarseness
- Children may only present with stridor or poor eating.

Does the pt have a history of foreign-body ingestions?
Psychiatric pts, prisoners, and children are more likely to ingest foreign bodies.

Has the pt had any bariatric surgery?
Gastric banding increases the risk of impaction of food boluses.

O — Evaluate pt's vital signs
Fever and hemodynamic instability may be seen with esophageal rupture.

Perform physical exam
General: Is the pt in distress? Able to swallow own secretions? Drooling? These are signs of severe distress.
HEENT: Perform a thorough inspection of the nose and mouth. Unilateral nasal discharge can be seen with nasal foreign bodies.
- Listen over trachea for stridor.

Lungs: Listen for wheezing or decreased breath sounds that may be seen with bronchial obstruction.
Abdomen: Generally normal. Note any tenderness, distention, or abnormal bowel sounds. Suggests bowel obstruction or perforation.

Obtain a CXR
Will show radio-opaque objects (e.g., button batteries, coins, dense plastic).

> - Coins will be seen on edge if in trachea or face on if in esophagus on posteroanterior CXR.

Mediastinal and/or subcutaneous air seen with esophageal perforation.

Obtain a lateral neck x-ray if proximal obstruction is suspected
CXR may miss objects in the posterior pharynx.

Consider a Gastrografin swallow
To demonstrate non-radiopaque objects

Consider direct laryngoscopy if pt feels the object in the upper airway
Allows direct visualization and removal.
Often, foreign-body sensation results from a small laceration or abrasion of the posterior pharynx caused by the foreign body (e.g., chicken bone).

Consider a chest and abdominal CT scan
Very sensitive in localizing foreign objects.
Can evaluate surrounding structures and may show alternative diagnosis.

A **Foreign-Body Ingestion**
Most common objects ingested are coins.
Objects tend to lodge at one of three levels:
- Cricopharyngeal level: Narrowest area in children. Can cause complete airway obstruction.
- T4 level: Aortic arch and carina. Most common in adults.
- Proximal to the gastroesophageal junction

Differential Diagnosis
Croup
Retropharyngeal abscess
Epiglottitis

P **Most objects that have passed into the stomach and small intestine can be observed and treated expectantly**
Arrange for emergent endoscopic removal of any foreign body causing obstruction or airway compromise
All button batteries in the esophagus need to be removed immediately. If the battery has passed into the stomach and intestine, it can be managed expectantly.
Sharp objects (e.g., knifes and glass) should be removed as soon as possible.

Schedule elective endoscopy for
Smooth objects in the esophagus that have not passed into the stomach after 24 hrs
Button batteries that have remained in the stomach more than 48 hrs

Food boluses can be treated with
IV glucagon: Can cause reflex contraction of the esophagus and expel the bolus.
Nitroglycerin/calcium channel blocker: Relax proximal gastroesophageal sphincter.
Do NOT treat with meat tenderizer because it may cause esophageal perforation.

Discharge pts
Who have had objects removed in the ED and have demonstrated that they can tolerate oral intake.
With objects that have passed into the small intestine. Instruct them to monitor their stool.
With button batteries in their stomach, but they will need to return within 48 hrs to ensure it has passed into the intestines.

Admit pts with
Esophageal foreign bodies or food boluses that cannot be treated in the ED

S What are the pt's symptoms?
Common symptoms include:
- Burning sensation in chest
- Nausea/vomiting
- Foul taste or odor in mouth

Atypical symptoms include:
- Hoarseness
- Shortness of breath
- Chronic cough
- Asthma

Do certain foods increase the symptoms?
Foods high in fat content or acidity tend to increase the symptoms.

Are the symptoms increased with certain positions?
Bending over or lying down tend to increase the symptoms.

Determine the pt's use or consumption of alcohol, tobacco, chocolate, or caffeine
All four of these products cause relaxation of the lower esophageal sphincter (LES), increasing gastroesophageal reflux disease (GERD) symptoms.

Has the pt tried any self-treatment?
Most pts will have already tried over-the-counter antacids, and their response to antacid treatment will help direct your treatment.

Has the pt experienced any dysphagia or odynophagia?
Dysphagia is suggestive of esophageal spasm or stricture.
Odynophagia is suggestive of ulcerative esophagitis.

Does the pt have any other medical problems?
History of coronary atherosclerotic disease (CAD) or risk factors for CAD may warrant cardiac workup because myocardial ischemia can present with symptoms consistent with GERD.

What medications is the pt taking?
Opiates, calcium channel blockers, nitrates, theophylline, and anticholinergics can all increase GERD symptoms by relaxing the LES.

O Perform a physical exam
Typically normal
Check rectal exam to rule out occult GI blood loss.

Consider obtaining an ECG
Rule out myocardial ischemia as cause of symptoms.

Consider obtaining the following labs
CBC: May see chronic anemia caused by esophagitis or peptic ulcer disease (PUD).
Cardiac enzymes: Evaluate for myocardial damage.

Consider obtaining a CXR
May demonstrate a hiatal hernia, although not all hiatal hernias cause symptoms.
Free air or pleural effusion may be seen with an esophageal perforation.
May see an esophageal foreign body.

A **Gastroesophageal Reflux Disease**
Syndrome caused by the reflux of gastric contents into the esophagus, causing local irritation and inflammation.

Differential Diagnosis
- Myocardial ischemia
- Cholelithiasis
- Gastroenteritis
- PUD
- Gastritis
- Esophageal foreign body

P **Give a trial of an antacid**
A GI cocktail consisting of viscous lidocaine, aluminum hydroxide/magnesium hydroxide, and Donnatal can provide almost immediate pain relief and improvement in symptoms.
Consider starting a proton pump inhibitor or histamine-2 receptor blocker.

Educate pt on lifestyle modifications
Elevate head of bed 4 inches.
Do not eat within 2 hrs of lying down.
Eat small meals and avoid overeating.
Avoid late-night meals or snacks.
Avoid foods that lower the LES tone (e.g., alcohol, caffeine, chocolate, or fatty foods).
Avoid medications that lower the LES tone.

Arrange outpatient evaluation
If diagnosis is unclear or pt has failed antacid treatment, consider:
- Endoscopy: Allows direct visualization of the esophageal and gastric mucosa. Helpful to rule out PUD.
- 24 esophageal pH probe: Highly sensitive to secure the diagnosis of chest pain caused by GERD. Not commonly performed, however, because endoscopy can usually make the diagnosis.

Most pts can be discharged home
Consider admission for any pt who has
Severe reactive airway disease
Dehydration
Evidence of esophageal perforation
Evidence of gastrointestinal bleed

S Has the pt noticed any bleeding?
GI bleeding may not be noticed, and the pt may only present with generalized weakness, fatigue, syncope, dyspnea on exertion, or lightheadedness.
Black, tarry stools or melena are commonly seen with upper GI bleeding.
Hematochezia (bloody diarrhea) can be seen with a brisk upper GI bleed or more commonly with a lower GI bleed.
Bright red blood on normal brown stool or on the toilet paper is common with anal fissures or hemorrhoids.
Coffee ground emesis may be seen with an upper GI bleed.

Does the pt have a history of peptic ulcer disease (PUD) or gastritis?
Increases risk for upper gastrointestinal bleeding

Does the pt have a history of diverticulosis?
Common in pts presenting with painless hematochezia, the hallmark of a diverticular bleed.

Has the pt been vomiting or retching a lot?
If bleeding follows the vomiting or retching, the cause is likely a Mallory-Weiss tear.

Has the pt been taking any medications?
Heavy NSAID or steroid use increases the risk for PUD and gastritis as the cause of an upper GI bleed.
Iron, bismuth, and charcoal can turn the stool black.

Has the pt recently undergone any endoscopic evaluation?
Ensure that pt is not having any postprocedural bleeding from polypectomy.

Does the pt drink large quantities of alcohol?
Suggests possibility of cirrhosis and secondary variceals as etiology of blood loss.

What other medical problems does the pt have?
Pt's with coronary atherosclerotic disease (CAD) are at risk for myocardial ischemia with severe anemia.

O Evaluate the pt's vital signs
Ensure that the pt is hemodynamically stable. Look for tachycardia and hypotension.

Perform a physical exam
Chest: Note any stigmata of liver disease (e.g., spider hemangiomas, gynecomastia).
Abdomen: May have tenderness to palpation. Note liver size to suggest cirrhosis.
Rectal: May note frank blood, hemocult-positive stool, or melena. Use anoscope to visualize internal hemorrhoids and anal fissures.

Perform a gastric lavage
Place a nasogastric (NG) tube and ensure that there is no blood with aspiration. Need to exclude an upper GI blood source and active bleeding.
Once lavage is performed, NG tube can be removed.

Obtain the following labs
CBC: Evaluate the degree of anemia. In an acute bleed, the hemoglobin may not equilibrate for several hours and is not indicative of actual blood loss.
- Note platelets and any thrombocytopenia.

PT, INR, PTT: Exclude coagulopathy as a confounding factor in the bleeding.
Type and cross: For PRBCs or clotting factors as needed.

Electrolytes, BUN, Creatinine: Exclude secondary metabolic disturbance or renal insufficiency.

Consider an ECG
Exclude cardiac ischemia with severe anemia.

A Gastrointestinal Bleeding
Upper sources:
- PUD
- Gastritis
- Esophageal varices
- Mallory-Weiss tear
- Angiodysplasia
- Esophagitis

Lower sources:
- Angiodysplasia
- Diverticular bleed
- Polyp or cancer
- Hemorrhoids
- Anal fissure

In pediatric pts, consider Meckel's diverticulum or intussusception.

Differential Diagnosis
- Acute abdomen
- Gastroesophageal reflux disease

P Start IV fluids
All pts should have two large-bore (> 16-gauge) peripheral IVs established. Maintain blood pressure with fluid boluses of crystalloid or colloid fluids.

Place on oxygen via nasal cannula
Helps improve oxygen delivery and prevent ischemia.

Transfuse PRBCs
If actively bleeding and Hg < 8 or < 10 with history of CAD or pt not responding to fluid boluses

Consult Gastroenterology
Consider emergent endoscopy to localize bleeding site and treat locally.

Consider Surgery consult for severe bleeding that may require surgical intervention
May need bleeding scan to localize bleeding.

Consider starting the following medications
Proton pump inhibitor/H_2 blocker: Decreases acid secretion and may prevent rebleeding with PUD and gastritis.
Vasopressin: Potent vasoconstrictor that may help decrease bleeding in variceal or ulcer bleeding.
Octreotide: Decreases recurrent variceal bleeding.

Follow serial hemoglobins.
Monitor for ongoing blood loss.

Most pts will be admitted
Admit all pts with ongoing blood loss or borderline vital signs to the ICU.

Discharge home pts who have
Stable vital signs, Hg > 10, no evidence of active bleeding, and normal coagulation studies

Hepatitis

S — What are the pt's current symptoms?
Common symptoms include:
- Malaise
- Lethargy
- Dark urine or stools
- RUQ pain
- Fever
- Jaundice

Less common symptoms include:
- Hepatic encephalopathy
- Edema
- Cirrhosis

Has the pt been vaccinated against Hepatitis A or B?
Hepatitis B vaccine will protect against Hepatitis B and D. A vaccine for Hepatitis A has been made available recently and is generally recommended for anyone who is going to travel.

Does the pt have any risk factors for hepatitis?
Viral Hepatitis B and C are associated with intravenous drug abuse, unprotected intercourse, tattoos, and blood transfusions.
Hepatitis A is associated with crowded conditions, poor sanitation, and recently several outbreaks have been attributed to green onions.

Has the pt been taking any medications?
Acetaminophen, isoniazid, methyldopa, and ketoconazole are just a few of the many medications associated with drug-induced hepatitis.
Review all medications, including chronic medications, because drug-induced hepatitis can occur at anytime.

Does the pt have a history of alcohol use?
Alcohol and viral hepatitis are the two most common causes in the United States.
May need to ask family members about the degree of alcohol use to get an accurate assessment.

Has the pt traveled recently? Does the pt work in a nursing home or day care facility?
Suggests Hepatitis A or E because of their spread through the fecal-oral route and association with poor sanitation.
If pt has been camping or hiking recently, ask about ingestion of any wild mushrooms (*Amanita* poisoning).

O — Perform a physical exam
HEENT: Scleral icterus? Icterus may be seen under the tongue. Nystagmus may be seen with encephalopathy.
Lungs: Typically normal, but may have dull breath sounds in the bases caused by pleural effusions.
Cardiac: Typically normal, but may have evidence of high-output cardiac failure caused by liver failure.
Chest: Spider angiomas?
Abdomen: Palpate liver; may note knobby texture. Note liver span (decreased in cirrhosis). Fluid wave? Ascites?
Rectal: Guaiac stool
Extremities: Asterixis? Palmar erythema?
Neurologic: Stuporous? Lethargic? Coma? Evaluate mental status.

Check the following labs
CBC: Rule out anemia. May also have an elevated WBC associated with infection.

BUN, Creatinine, Electrolytes, LFT: Evaluate renal function. May see electrolyte disturbances, and elevations in LFT. End-stage hepatitis may have normal LFT.
- AST/ALT > 2 suggests alcohol liver disease.
- Albumin and total bilirubin evaluate the synthetic function of the liver.

Ammonia level: Can be followed clinically to assess liver function. Level does not correlate to the degree of encephalopathy present.
Coagulation studies: PT may be elevated when liver synthetic function is suppressed.
Acetaminophen level: Exclude acetaminophen toxicity.
Hepatitis serologies:
- HAV: IgM and IgG for HAV. IgM elevation consistent with acute illness.
- HBV: HBs antibody seen with immunization. HBc antibody, HBs antigen, and HBe antigen seen with HBV infection. HBe antigen associated with high infectivity.
- HCV: Check HCV IgG.

A Hepatitis
Etiologies can be from alcohol, viruses (Hepatitis A, B, C, D, E, cytomegalovirus, Epstein-Barr virus, herpes simplex virus), toxic exposure (halothane), or drug use. Chronic hepatitis exists after 6 months of symptoms or persistent lab abnormalities. Acute hepatitis < 6 months.

Differential Diagnosis
- Cholecystitis - Biliary cirrhosis
- Cholangitis   - Steatohepatitis

P Provide supportive care
Consider IV hydration and antiemetics.

Stop any potentially hepatotoxic medications or drugs
Avoid prescribing any hepatotoxic medications (e.g., acetaminophen).

Consider contact prophylaxis for Hepatitis A or B
Immune globulin plus vaccination if exposure has been recent.

Treat any coagulopathies with fresh frozen plasma or vitamin K
Start lactulose if hepatic encephalopathy present
Consider paracentesis in any pt with ascites and fever
Exclude spontaneous bacterial peritonitis.

Disposition
Most pts will need to be admitted for IV hydration and further evaluation.
Consider discharge only in those pts with mild symptoms, mild laboratory abnormalities, and who can have close follow-up arranged.
Pts with hepatic encephalopathy, major coagulopathies, or gastrointestinal bleeding will need to be admitted to the ICU.

Ischemic Bowel

S

What are the pt's current symptoms?
The classic description is abdominal pain out of proportion to the exam.
Common symptoms include:
- Abdominal pain
- Nausea/Vomiting
- Diarrhea
- GI bleeding

May see:
- Mental status changes
- Fever
- Syncope

Does the pt note anything that exacerbates the pain?
Chronic bowel ischemia typically presents as dull, crampy, postprandial abdominal pain caused by a narrowing in the celiac or superior mesenteric arteries from atherosclerosis.

Does the pt have any risk factors for vascular disease?
- Diabetes
- Peripheral vascular disease
- Tobacco use
- Hypercholesterolemia
- Coronary atherosclerotic disease
- Increases risk for ischemia bowel

What other medical conditions does the pt have?
Helpful to ascertain risk factors and other etiologies for presenting complaints. Bowel ischemia can be seen post–myocardial infarction (MI) and with congestive heart failure (CHF), when cardiac output is low enough to cause ischemia.

O

Evaluate the pt's vital signs
Perform a physical exam
HEENT, Lungs, Cardiac: Typically normal. May see signs of CHF.
Abdomen: Peritoneal signs? Tenderness? Listen for bruits.
Rectal: Guaiac stool. Guaiac-positive stool seen with ischemic bowel.
Neurologic: Note any mental status changes.

Obtain the following labs
CBC: May have elevated WBC. Exclude anemia.
BUN, Creatinine, LFT, Amylase, Lipase, Electroytes: Exclude alternative diagnosis.
- May see elevations in liver enzymes caused by hepatic ischemia.
- Typically will have a metabolic acidosis.

Lactic acid level: Very sensitive for ischemia, although not specific for bowel ischemia.

Consider obtaining abdominal x-rays
Useful to exclude free air and bowel obstruction. Used less frequently now with CT scans so readily available.

Consider an abdominal CT scan
May be normal initially. Bowel wall thickening, streaking of mesenteric fat, and loss of IV contrast in the celiac or superior mesenteric artery can make the diagnosis.

Consider an angiogram
The gold standard in making the diagnosis of arterial insufficiency. May also be therapeutic because an interventional radiologist can open an obstruction with balloon angioplasty or an injection of papaverine.

Consider colonoscopy or sigmoidoscopy
Allows direct visualization of the colon, which will display ischemic changes.

A Ischemic Bowel
Caused by subacute closure or thrombosis of the celiac, superior mesenteric, or inferior mesenteric arteries (IMA). The IMA supplies the left colon and rectum and has adequate collateral support from the rectal blood supply, so it is not typically associated with ischemic bowel.

Acute presentations are typically the result of embolic events or as a result of inadequate blood flow caused by CHF, aortic dissection, hypotension, sepsis, or MI.

Chronic presentations (intestinal angina) are caused by atherosclerosis of the blood supply and typically present with postprandial pain.

Differential Diagnosis
- Intestinal obstruction
- Cholelithiasis
- Volvulus
- Pancreatitis
- Intussusception
- Abdominal aortic aneurysm
- Aortic dissection

P Initiate supportive care
Ensure adequate blood pressure.
- Hydrate with normal saline solution. Pt may require large volumes of fluid replacement.
- Avoid pressors if possible because they may exacerbate the ischemia.

Treat any underlying disorder (e.g., CHF, MI, aortic dissection) that may have incited the ischemia.

Provide adequate pain relief
Pain is typically out of proportion to the exam; however, this should not limit narcotic use.

Consider starting IV antibiotics
In order to prevent secondary infection from translocation of bowel flora

Consult a general surgeon for possible surgical correction
Interventional radiology consult should also be considered for angiogram and possible balloon angioplasty.

Disposition
All pts should be admitted.
Consider ICU admission for any pt showing any signs of hypotension or hypovolemia.

Mortality rate is 50% to 100% without aggressive treatment and repair.

Pancreatitis

S — What are the pt's symptoms?
Common symptoms include:
- Midepigastric abdominal pain
- Anorexia
- Nausea/Vomiting
- Distention

Has the pt noticed anything that exacerbates the pain?
Pain typically increases several hours after eating, and may increase with lying down.

Does anything help alleviate the pain?
Pain typically decreases if the pt avoids eating/drinking or leans forward.

Does the pt have any risk factors for pancreatitis?
- Alcohol use
- Hypertriglycerides
- Peptic ulcer disease
- Cholelithiasis
- Scorpion bite
- Recent endoscopic retrograde cholangiopancreatography (ERCP)

Does the pt take any medications or herbal supplements?
Oral contraceptives, diuretics, steroids, and aspirin are a few drugs associated with pancreatitis.

Does the pt have any other medical problems?
Pts with a history of pancreatitis may not demonstrate elevations of amylase and lipase. Pancreatitis is associated with cystic fibrosis, lupus, and recent abdominal surgery. Consider a retained common bile duct stone as a cause in anyone who has had a cholecystectomy in the last 2 years.

Obtain a social history
Alcohol use and cholelithiasis are the two leading causes of pancreatitis in the United States.

O — Perform a physical exam
HEENT, Lungs, Cardiac: Typically normal.
Abdomen: Tenderness? Peritoneal signs?

- *Grey-Turner's sign*: Ecchymosis along the flank caused by retroperitoneal hemorrhage.
- *Cullen's sign*: Ecchymosis around the umbilicus caused by intraperitoneal hemorrhage.

Rectal: Exclude gastrointestinal bleeding.

Obtain the following labs
CBC: Exclude anemia or elevated WBC.
BUN, Creatinine, Electrolytes: Exclude an underlying renal or electrolyte disturbance.
LFT, amylase, lipase: Amylase and lipase are typically elevated in acute pancreatitis, although they may be normal in chronic pancreatitis.
- Lipase is more sensitive and specific for pancreas injury.
- May see elevated alkaline phosphatase, and bilirubin to suggest gallstones.
- Elevations in AST > ALT seen with alcohol abuse.

ESR, CRP: Signs of inflammation and may be elevated in chronic pancreatitis despite having normal amylase and lipase.

Consider abdominal CT scan
Can demonstrate edema and/or necrosis of the pancreas. Calcification and atrophy of the pancreas seen in chronic pancreatitis.

Consider RUQ ultrasound
Poor sensitivity for evaluating the pancreas but useful to rule out cholelithiasis.

A Pancreatitis
Inflammation of the pancreas that is associated with edema, autodigestion, necrosis, and possible hemorrhage.
Chronic pancreatitis can lead to diabetes.
Ranson's criteria can help predict overall mortality.
- Initial criteria include:
  - Age > 55
  - WBC > 16,000
  - Glucose > 200
  - LDH > 350
  - AST > 250
- Criteria after 48 hours:
  - HCT ↓ by 10%
  - BUN ↑ by 5 mg/dL
  - Calcium < 8 mg/dL
  - PaO_2 < 60 mm Hg
  - Base Deficit > 4
  - Fluid Deficit > 6 L
  - Mortality nearly 100% if > 6 criteria are seen.

Differential Diagnosis
- Peptic ulcer disease
- Abdominal aortic aneurysm
- Renal colic
- Cholelithiasis
- Ischemic bowel
- Intestinal obstruction

P Provide supportive care
Pts may require aggressive IV hydration because of fluid sequestration and third spacing.
Keep pt NPO until pain has resolved.
- May give trial of clear liquids for mild disease.

Provide adequate pain control with narcotics.
Treat nausea and vomiting with antiemetics.

Treat underlying disorder if possible
Pts with retained gallstones may require surgery or ERCP to decompress the biliary and pancreatic system.
Withhold any medications or alcohol that may have caused the pancreatitis.

Consider starting antibiotics
Imipenem has been shown to decrease mortality in necrotizing pancreatitis.

Disposition
Most pts will need to be admitted for IV hydration and pain control.
- Consider ICU admission for pts who present with hypotension, have multiple comorbid illnesses, or have multiple Ranson's criteria because pancreatitis can progress quickly to multiorgan system failure and death.

Consider discharging home any pts who are able to tolerate clear liquids in the ED, able to adequately hydrate themselves, have mild disease, and have close follow-up arranged.

Peptic Ulcer Disease — Gastrointestinal

S **What are the pt's current symptoms?**
Common symptoms include:
- Epigastric abdominal pain
- Heartburn
- Nausea/Vomiting
- Melena
- Early satiety
- Bloating

May complain of:
- Hematemesis
- Hematochezia
- Fatigue
- Lethargy

Does the pt have a history of heartburn or peptic ulcer disease (PUD)?
Determine whether the pt's present symptoms are different or whether this is a flare-up.

How are the pt's symptoms related to eating?
Gastric ulcer pain typically occurs immediately after eating.
Duodenal ulcer pain typically occurs 1 to 3 hrs after eating.

What medications is the pt taking?
NSAIDs and steroids increase the risk for PUD.
Medication profile is also helpful to see what medications (e.g., over-the-counter antacids) the pt has tried to alleviate symptoms.

What other medical problems does the pt have?
Helps to exclude other etiologies for the pt's symptoms.
PUD is also associated with renal failure, inflammatory bowel disease (e.g., Crohn's disease), and autoimmune disorders that frequently require NSAID or steroid use.

Obtain a social history
Tobacco and alcohol use increase the risk for PUD.

O **Evaluate the pt's vital signs**
Tachycardia and hypotension suggests blood loss or severe dehydration.

Perform a physical exam
HEENT, Lungs, Cardiac: Typically normal.
Abdomen: Epigastric tenderness may be present. Severe pain suggests perforation.
Rectal: Guaiac positive? Seen with PUD. Frank blood? Suggests a severe bleed.

Obtain the following labs
CBC to exclude anemia.
Electroytes, LFT, amylase, lipase to exclude other causes of abdominal pain.
Coagulation studies to exclude a coagulopathy.

Consider sending a Type and Screen/Cross if there are signs/symptoms of recent blood loss

Consider sending *Helicobacter pylori* testing
IgG serology can be sent to see if pt warrants treatment.

Consider obtaining a CXR
Exclude free air secondary to perforation.

Place a nasogastric tube if there has been any hematemesis or hematochezia
Exclude any active upper gastrointestinal bleeding.

Peptic Ulcer Disease

Consider emergent endoscopy if active bleeding is noted
Can be diagnostic and therapeutic.

A **Peptic Ulcer Disease**

Helicobacter pylori, a urease-producing gram-negative rod, is the most common cause of PUD.
- Disrupts the mucosal protective barrier of the stomach and duodenum.
- Responsible for approximately 95% of gastric ulcers and 85% of duodenal ulcers.

Rare causes include Zollinger-Ellison syndrome and gastrinomas.

Differential Diagnosis
- Acute gastritis
- Cholecystitis
- Abdominal obstruction
- Pancreatitis
- Gastroesophageal reflux disease
- Ischemic bowel
- Hepatitis

P **Provide supportive care**
Provide IV hydration and pain control.
Consider a trial of a GI cocktail (i.e., viscous lidocaine, Donnatal, aluminum hydroxide/magnesium hydroxide).

Consider obtaining a gastroenterology consult
For emergent endoscopy if there are signs of active blood loss

Educate the pt on lifestyle changes to include
- Bland diet
- Avoid aspirin, NSAIDs
- Small meals
- Alcohol and tobacco avoidance

Start a proton pump inhibitor, H_2 blocker, or sucralfate
Decreases acid secretion, allowing the gastric and duodenal mucosa to heal more rapidly.

Consider starting treatment for *Helicobacter pylori*
Multiple regimens have been shown to be effective.
Treatment of *H. pylori* has been shown to decrease ulcer recurrence to less than 10%.

Disposition
Most pts can be discharged home with routine follow-up with their primary care provider.
Admit any pt with evidence of blood loss, severe symptoms, persistent vomiting, or evidence of perforation.

VI
HEENT

Conjunctivitis

S **What are the pt's current symptoms?**
Common symptoms include:
- Red eye
- Blurred vision
- Increased lacrimation
- Pain
- Discharge
- Photophobia

Does the pt wear contact lenses?
Contact lens wearers are at increased risk for pseudomonas conjunctivitis and corneal ulcers.
Inadequate rinsing of the lens before insertion can also cause chemical conjunctivitis.

Has the pt been around anyone else with similar symptoms?
Viruses (e.g., adenovirus) are the most common cause of conjunctivitis. Viral infections are easily transmissible.

Does the pt suffer from seasonal allergies or hay fever?
Suggest allergic conjunctivitis, which commonly affects both eyes, as opposed to one seen with infectious conjunctivitis.

Has the pt noticed any rashes or pain before current symptoms?
A preceding rash or pain suggests a zoster infection.

Does the pt have any other medical problems?
Exclude any immunosuppressed states that place the pt at risk for a fungal infection.

What medications has the pt been using?
Inquire specifically about any eye drops or ointments.
Sulfacetamide is an eye drop or ointment that commonly causes increased redness and eye irritation with use.

Obtain a social history to include a sexual history
Gonorrhea or chlamydia can cause aggressive eye infections.
Obtain an occupational history.
- Metal or wood workers are at increased risk for occult foreign bodies in the eye.
- Welders can suffer from corneal abrasions and flash burns if they do not wear the proper eye protection ALL of the time.

Obtain a review of symptoms
May help elicit another cause for the pt's current symptoms.

O **Perform a physical exam**
Eye Exam:
- Evaluate and document visual acuity.
- Measure intraocular pressure with tonometry.
  - Done to exclude glaucoma.
  - Acute onset of glaucoma can present with red eye and lead rapidly to permanent blindness.
- Perform fundoscopic exam. You may need to dilate the pupil to get an adequate exam.
- Perform slit lamp exam. Be sure to invert eyelids to look for foreign bodies.
  - Stain both eyes with fluorescein and note any uptake.
    - Corneal abrasion will appear as pooling of the fluorescein.
    - Corneal ulcers appear white or hazy.
    - Dendritic-shaped uptake seen in herpes.
  - Note any anterior chamber inflammation or flare cells.

HEENT: Note any lymphadenopathy, otitis externa or media, or rashes.
- Note any signs of periorbital cellulites.

Consider sending bacterial cultures on any purulent exudates

A **Conjunctivitis**
Inflammation of the conjunctiva caused by infection or chemical or allergic reaction. History and physical most helpful in determining underlying cause of symptoms. Most common eye infection. Can be caused by viruses, bacteria, or fungus.

Differential Diagnosis
- Glaucoma
- Corneal abrasion
- Iritis
- Orbital cellulitis
- Periorbital cellulitis

P **Treatment based on cause of conjunctivitis**
General: Supportive care with cool compresses and ocular decongestants (e.g., tetrahydrozoline or naphazoline). Educate pt to wash hands frequently in order to prevent spread. Contact lenses should not be worn for 7 days to prevent corneal ulcers.
Viral: No specific treatment needed. A self-limited illness. Antibiotic drops and ointments are commonly prescribed, but there is no evidence that they provide any benefit.
Bacterial: Topical antibiotic ointment or drops for at least 5 days. Antibiotic should have antipseudomonal coverage if pt wears contact lenses.
Gonorrhea/Chlamydia: If suspected, treat the pt with systemic antibiotics.
Herpes: Treat with systemic antivirals. Ensure pt has close follow-up with ophthalmologist.
Allergic: Consider systemic antihistamines, along with ocular antihistamines.

Disposition
Most pts will be able to be discharged home.
Admission should be considered in pts with severe herpes infections, severe corneal abrasions, or gonorrhea infection.

Corneal Abrasion

S

What are the pt's current symptoms?
Typical symptoms include:
- Pain
- Photophobia
- Red eye
- Increased lacrimation
- Sensation of foreign body

Does the pt remember scratching or getting something in the eye?
It is not uncommon for there to be no history of a foreign body.

Does the pt wear contact lenses?
Increases risk for pseudomonas infections and corneal ulcers.

What kind of work does the pt do?
Wood or metal workers are at increased risk for foreign bodies.
- Be sure to ask about any hobbies the pt has because metal working might not be the primary profession.
- Ask specifically about grinding metal because this is a high-speed injury, where metal particles can be injected into the globe of the eye.
- Document whether the pt uses eye protection.

Welders are at increased risk for UV keratitis.

Has the pt been a victim of any trauma?
A blow to the eye can result in a hyphema or traumatic iritis, causing similar symptoms.

Document tetanus status
What self-treatment has the pt done before coming to the ED?
Inquire about flushing eyes, medication used, or any attempts at removing foreign bodies.

What medical problems does the pt have?
Exclude immunosuppressive states or coagulopathies that may exacerbate the condition.

Obtain a social history
Inquire about hobbies such as using tanning booths or recent exposure to prolonged sunlight, which increases risk for UV keratitis.

O

Evaluate the pt's vital signs
Include visual acuity with and without correction as a vital sign.

Perform a physical exam
Eye:
- Evaluate extraocular movement.
- Visually inspect for foreign body.
  - Rust rings may be noted if metallic foreign bodies are present.
  - Invert eyelids to look for hidden foreign bodies.
- Instill fluorescein and note any pooling consistent with corneal abrasion.
- Perform slit lamp exam and note any signs of inflammation or abrasions.
- Perform tonometry to exclude glaucoma. Do not test if there is evidence of a corneal laceration or globe rupture.

HEENT: Note any signs of trauma, burns, or infection.

Consider x-ray or CT scan of orbits
Useful to exclude intraocular foreign bodies or posterior eye injuries.
Can also be used to exclude fractures.

HEENT

A — Corneal Abrasion
Epithelial defect of the cornea

Differential Diagnosis
Traumatic iritis: Inflammation of the iris, typically from blunt trauma
Ultraviolet keratitis: Radiation injury of the cornea caused by welding, sunlight, or tanning booths
Hyphema: Blood in the anterior chamber arising from the iris or ciliary body. Usually the result of a direct blow.

P

Provide effective pain relief
Topical anesthetics can provide immediate relief and allow painless removal of a foreign body.
- Do not discharge pt with topical anesthetics because it can inhibit healing and allow further damage of the cornea from repetitive injury that is missed with loss of sensation.

Topical NSAIDs, cycloplegics, and narcotic pain medicine can be effective in providing pain relief.

Remove the foreign body
Foreign-body removal can be done with irrigation, cotton-tipped applicator, needle, or high-speed burr.
Rust rings must be removed, although removal can be delayed until the next day when pt is able to be seen by an ophthalmologist.

Irrigate the eye until eye pH is normal
If pt has had a chemical exposure to the eye
Most important with alkaline (e.g., lyme) injuries because these penetrate deeply into the eye and can be much more destructive.

Consider antibiotic ointment/drops
All contact lens wearers should receive antipseudomonal antibiotic coverage and be advised not to wear their contact lenses until symptoms have completely resolved.
Antibiotic ointments or drops are commonly prescribed, although there is no evidence that they improve outcomes or expedite healing.

Limit use of eye patches
They hinder depth perception and have not been shown to aid in healing.

S What are the pt's current symptoms?
Common symptoms include:
- Difficulty swallowing liquids or solids
- Having to turn head/neck in order to swallow
- Sensation of food sticking
- Chest pain
- Pain with swallowing (odynophagia)

Does the pt have trouble initiating the swallowing reflex or feel like food is getting stuck?
Trouble initiating the swallowing reflex suggests a problem with a cranial nerve.
- May complain of having to try to swallow multiple times before successful.
- Cranial nerves V, IX, X, XI, and XII all play a role in swallowing.

Food getting stuck suggests an esophageal disorder secondary to spasm or a motility disorder.

What is the pt able to swallow?
Solid food is typically worse than liquids with esophageal disorders, but liquids are worse with cranial nerve disorders.
Ensure that pt is able to swallow own secretions.

Has the pt choked on anything or is there a history of foreign-body ingestion?
An impacted food bolus or foreign body may need to be removed endoscopically.
Ingestion of a button battery requires emergent removal if it is lodged in the esophagus.

What other medical conditions does the pt have?
Dysphagia caused by esophageal spasm can be seen with diabetes, gastroesophageal reflux disease (GERD), and connective tissue disorders.
Amyloidosis can cause thickening of the esophagus and limit peristalsis.

Obtain a social history
Alcohol use can cause esophageal spasm and increased risk for peptic ulcer disease and GERD.

O Evaluate the pt's vital signs
Ensure that vitals are stable and pt is not in respiratory distress.

Perform a physical exam
Typically normal
HEENT: May note gagging or drooling. Carefully examine mouth and evaluate pt's ability to swallow.
Lungs: Egophony? Wheezing? May be noted with aspiration.
Neurologic: Do a detailed cranial nerve exam. Note movement and strength of tongue, ability to elevate soft palate, ability to swallow, and sensation to face and tongue.

Obtain x-rays
CXRs may show foreign bodies, pneumonia, masses, or lack of air in stomach.
Neck x-rays may be needed to exclude foreign bodies.

Consider obtaining an ECG
If pt has associated chest pain

Dysphagia

Laboratory studies are generally not helpful

Consider obtaining a GI consult for urgent endoscopy
Endoscopy allows direct visualization of the esophagus and can be therapeutic with removal of foreign bodies.

A — Dysphagia
Difficulty swallowing caused by esophageal or oropharyngeal disorders
May be a symptom of another disease process, such as:
- Cerebrovascular accident
- Sjogren's syndrome
- Esophagitis
- Achalasia
- Foreign-body ingestion
- Myasthenia gravis
- GERD
- Diabetes
- Multiple sclerosis

P — Ensure that airway is protected because pts are at risk for aspiration

Provide supportive care
IV hydration
Pain control

If there is a suspected foreign body or food bolus, consider
IV or IM glucagon: Can help increase peristalsis and ejection of the foreign body.
Calcium channel blockers or nitroglycerin: Can relax the smooth muscle of the esophagus and may help the foreign body pass into the stomach.
Gastroenterology consult for urgent endoscopy for direct visualization and removal
- A must if the foreign body is a button battery.

Disposition
Discharge pts who have had foreign bodies removed or symptoms relieved with treatment and who have been observed to eat and drink without difficulty.
- All pts should have close follow-up with their primary care provider or a gastroenterologist.

Admit pts who are unable to drink liquids safely or who are at high risk for aspiration.

S Does the pt have a history of nosebleeds?
Does the pt know what causes the nosebleeds?
Has the pt ever had to have the nose packed or cauterized?
- Helpful to determine the severity of past nosebleeds.

Has there been any trauma?
Specifically ask about localized trauma from nose picking.

Does the pt suffer from allergies?
Recurrent epistaxis is associated with dry mucosal membranes caused by allergies.

In children, specifically inquire about the possibility of a foreign body
What type of heat does the pt have in the home?
Forced-air heat is associated with drier air and can lead to dry mucosal membranes and epistaxis. Less of an issue with radiators.

What medical problems does the pt have?
Epistaxis has been associated with uncontrolled hypertension.
History of coagulopathies or use of blood thinners increases the severity of epistaxis.

What medications does the pt take?
Inquire specifically about warfarin, aspirin, clopidogrel, and other blood thinners.

Obtain a social history
Snorting of drugs, in particular cocaine, can cause septal perforations and bleeding.
Heavy alcohol use can cause thrombocytopenia and coagulopathies, increasing the severity of the epistaxis.

O Evaluate the pt's vital signs
Ensure that pt is not orthostatic from severe blood loss.

Perform a physical exam
HEENT: Visually inspect the nose.
- Most bleeding arises from Kiesselbach's plexus along the anterior nasal septum.
- Depending on the degree of bleeding, you may need to pack the nose with gauze treated with lidocaine and neosynephrine to cause vasoconstriction and slow the bleeding.
- If no bleeding is seen anterior but there is active bleeding, the source is typically posterior and will require nasal packing.

Consider sending the following labs
CBC: Evaluate degree of blood loss and obtain baseline if there has been significant bleeding. Exclude thrombocytopenia.
Coagulation studies: Ascertain whether there is a coagulopathy.
Type and screen: If blood products will need to be administered.

Consider facial x-rays or CT scan if bleeding is caused by trauma
Exclude facial fracture.

A Epistaxis
Nose bleeding that can be from the anterior or posterior portion of the nose
- Approximately 90% of epistaxis is from anterior sources, in particular Kiesselbach's plexus. Usually a self-limited process that is easily treated in the ED.
- Posterior epistaxis tends to be much more serious and arises from larger vessels. Can result in significant blood loss and is much more difficult to control in the ED.

Differential Diagnosis
- Hypertension
- Anticoagulant therapy
- Foreign body
- Cocaine use

P General treatment principles
All pts should be encouraged to use a humidifier at home to prevent dry mucous membranes.
Encourage use of normal saline nasal sprays.
Advise pts to avoid aspirin, NSAIDs, and any activities that can increase intranasal pressure, such as bending over, sneezing, or nose blowing.

Provide hemostasis by
Anterior epistaxis:
- Hold direct pressure for 15 minutes.
- Consider neosynephrine topical use to constrict blood vessels.
- Consider cauterization with silver nitrate after providing anesthesia with topical lidocaine if the bleeding site can be directly visualized.
- If above measure fails, the nose will need to be packed. Numerous systems are available for nasal packings, and it is important to become familiar with your particular system before needing to use it.
  - Place all pts with nasal packings on antistaphylococcus antibiotics to prevent toxic shock syndrome.
  - All pts with nasal packing need to be evaluated by ENT within 3 days to have packing removed.

Posterior epistaxis:
- Difficult to hold direct pressure, so this step is usually futile.
- Consider packing the nose with gauze soaked in neosynephrine and lidocaine.
- Above measures are typically unsuccessful. Nasal packing with a balloon tamponade device is generally required.
  - Start pt on antistaphylococcus antibiotics.
  - Most pts will need to be admitted or arranged to follow up with ENT in the a.m.

Otitis Externa

S — **What are the pt's current symptoms?**
Common symptoms include:
- Ear pain
- Discharge
- Decreased hearing
- Headache

Does the pt have a history of recurrent otitis externa?
Helpful to determine whether the recurrences are a result of reinfection or inadequate treatment.

Does the pt swim, take baths, or use a hot tub frequently?
Increases susceptibility to otitis externa (swimmer's ear).

Does the pt have a history of diabetes?
Malignant otitis externa is a pseudomonas infection that starts as an otitis externa and extends into the mastoid air cells. Most commonly associated with diabetes and immunosuppressed states.

Has there been any trauma?
Exclude cerebrospinal leak caused by basal skull fracture as cause of ear drainage.

What has the pt tried at home to treat self?
Helps direct your treatment.

Is there any possibility of a foreign body?
Cotton-tipped applicator swabs can break off and cause infection.
Insects can cause pain and a localized reaction.
Children are known to put things into their ears that can cause pain and discharge days or weeks later.

What medical problems does the pt have?
May help elicit an immunocompromised state or alternative diagnosis.

O — **Perform a physical exam**
Ear:
- Perform visual inspection of external ear and canal. Note any battle signs, discharge, tenderness, or erythema.
- Visualize tympanic membrane. Remove cerumen if necessary.
- Note any tenderness over the mastoid process.
- Note any lymphadenopathy.

Complete a full HEENT exam.
Neurologic: Note any cranial nerve deficits. Pay particular attention to cranial nerves V and VII.

Consider obtaining the following labs
CBC: WBC may be elevated in malignant otitis externa.
ESR: Significant elevation suggests malignant otitis externa.

Consider obtaining a head CT to include temporal bones
Can see diagnostic changes to make the diagnosis of malignant otitis externa.

HEENT

A. Otitis Externa
Infection of the external ear or auditory canal

-or-

Malignant Otitis Externa
Infection that starts in the external ear or auditory canal and extends into adjacent tissues.
An aggressive infection that is more common in diabetics.
Can lead to cranial nerve deficits, permanent hearing loss, and meningitis.

Differential Diagnosis
- Cerumen impaction
- Foreign body

P. Otitis Externa
Can be quite painful, and it is not uncommon for pts to require narcotic pain relief.
Treat infection with topical antibiotics.
- Consider placing a wick if difficult to instill antibiotic drops with swelling present.
- Antibiotic of choice is corticosporin otic suspension or a fluoroquinolone.
  - Limit use of corticosporin otic solution to situations where you can guarantee that the tympanic membrane is intact because the solution is toxic to the middle ear.

Educate pt on how to clean the ear with hydrogen peroxide.
Most pts can be discharged home with follow-up with their primary care provider.

Malignant Otitis Externa
Most pts will need to be admitted for IV antibiotics and possible debridement.
Start antipseudomonas antibiotics in the ED.
- Will require double coverage for pseudomonas.

Send a bacterial culture of any discharge present.
Consider ENT consult for possible debridement.
Ensure that diabetes is adequately controlled to facilitate clearance of the infection.

S — What are the pt's current symptoms?
Common symptoms include:
- Ear pain
- Fever
- Decreased hearing
- Headache

In children, may see:
- Increased irritability
- Vomiting
- Anorexia

Does the pt have a history of recurrent ear infections?
Recurrent infections can be caused by anatomic abnormalities or eustachian tube dysfunction.

Inquire as to whether the pt has ever had "tubes" placed in the ears and when was the last time.
- Tympanostomy tubes have been shown to significantly reduce the incidence of otitis media.

If a child, is the pt exposed to second-hand smoke?
Exposure to second-hand smoke has been shown to increase the incidence of otitis media and asthma exacerbations.

Has the pt been on antibiotics recently?
Often, pts are started on antibiotic treatment by their primary care provider (PCP)/pediatrician and present to the ED later complaining of continued symptoms that have not resolved with treatment.

If pt has been on amoxicillin, check to see if it was low dose (40 mg/kg divided) or high dose (80 mg/kg divided). Pts may fail treatment with low dose and be successfully treated with high dose, without a need to add a new antibiotic.

What other medical problems does the pt have?
Ear pain can be a sign of seasonal allergies with eustachian tube dysfunction and increased middle ear pressure without any infection.

What medications is the pt taking?
Ask about over-the-counter medications that may have already been tried. It is important to ask about dose and frequency because pts/parents tend to underdose.

O — Evaluate the pt's vital signs
Temperature higher than 40°C suggests a complicated infection or an additional infectious source.

Perform a physical exam
HEENT:
- Visualize the external ear and auditory canal. Note any erythema, swelling, or tenderness.
- Visualize the entire tympanic membrane (TM). Remove cerumen if necessary. Note whether the membrane is bulging, retracted, red, opacified, or perforated.
  - In children, it is important to perform pneumatic otoscopy because lack of movement of the TM is the most sensitive finding in otitis media.
  - Bulging TM is seen with acute otitis media.
  - Retracted TM is seen with chronic otitis media.
- Inspect the pharynx because pharyngeal edema can lead to eustachian tube dysfunction and ear pain.
- Complete a full HEENT exam.

Lungs: Note any wheezing or egophony, decreased breath sounds that might support an associated pneumonia.

No labs or x-rays are generally needed
Consider checking CXR, CBC, or urinalysis if temperature is greater than 40°C to exclude an additional infectious source.

A ### Otitis Media
An infection of the middle ear most commonly seen in children between the ages of 6 to 18 months and 4 to 5 years old (secondary to starting school).

Differential Diagnosis
- Otitis externa
- Foreign body
- Barotrauma to TM
- TM perforation
- Cerumen impaction

P ### Start oral antibiotic therapy
High-dose amoxicillin, oral cephalosporin, TMP-SMX, macrolide, or IM ceftriaxone

Consider starting a decongestant
Oral decongestants may reduce edema and improve eustachian tube function.

Consider pain relievers
Narcotics are often needed to control the intense pain associated with otitis media.

Educate parents on proper ibuprofen and acetaminophen dosing for the treatment of fever or pain
Disposition
Most pts can be discharged home with follow-up with their PCP/pediatricians. Admit pts who are dehydrated and unable to tolerate oral hydration or medications.

Pharyngitis — HEENT

S — **What are the pt's current symptoms?**
Common symptoms for pharyngitis include:
- Throat pain
- Odynophagia
- Headache
- Fever
- Cough
- Rhinorrhea

Symptoms seen with a peritonsillar abscess include:
- Hoarseness
- Trismus
- Muffled or hot potato voice

Symptoms seen with a retropharyngeal abscess include:
- Chest pain
- Neck pain
- Typically will not have trismus

Has the pt had upper respiratory infection symptoms (e.g., cough, rhinorrhea)?
Seen more commonly with viral illnesses, although pts can have secondary bacterial infections.

Has the pt been exposed to anyone with strep throat?
Can be transferred to close contacts by sharing eating utensils or intimate contact.

Are the pt's vaccinations up-to-date?
Ask specifically about the *Haemophilus influenzae* vaccine.

- Since the introduction of the HIB vaccine, epiglottitis is rare in children, but it is becoming an increasingly more common adult disease.

Does the pt have any other medical problems?
Any immunosuppressive disorder (e.g., chronic steroid use for chronic obstructive pulmonary disease/asthma, diabetes) can increase the pt's risk for a retropharyngeal abscess or peritonsillar abscess.

What medications does the pt take?
Inquire about recent antibiotic use because it will affect your management at discharge.

Obtain a social history
Obtain a sexual history because persistent pharyngitis can be caused by chlamydia or gonorrhea infections and is often missed on the initial presentation.

Obtain a review of symptoms
Ask specifically about penile discharge, dysuria, or polyuria if pt is sexually active and you suspect the pharyngitis is from an STD.

O — **Evaluate the pt's vital signs**
Perform a physical exam
General: Toxic appearance and respiratory compromise should suggest a retropharyngeal or peritonsillar abscess.
- If you suspect epiglottitis, do not agitate the child and allow him or her to assume any position of comfort.

HEENT: Perform a thorough inspection of the pharynx.
- Note any swelling or exudates of the tonsillar pillars.
- Note any deviation of the uvula or unilateral swelling of the peritonsillar space.
  ◆ Seen with peritonsillar abscess.
- On neck exam, note any swelling or lymphadenopathy.

Consider sending the following labs
Rapid strep test: Antigen test for group B strep that returns in about 15 minutes.
Throat culture: More sensitive than the rapid strep test for group B strep.
Gonorrhea/Chlamydia cultures: If you suspect an STD-related pharyngitis.

Consider obtaining the following radiology studies
Lateral x-ray of the neck:
- May demonstrate edema of the epiglottis and the classic thumbprint sign.
- May see prevertebral edema and air with a retropharyngeal abscess.

Neck CT scan:
- Imaging study of choice for evaluation of the soft tissue structures of the pharynx and larynx. If concerned about submandibular abscess (Lugwig's angina), be sure to order the scan to extend into the chest because these infections can extend along the fascial planes into the mediastinum.

A

Pharyngitis
Inflammation/infection of the pharynx and tonsils

Retropharyngeal Abscess
Typically occurs in children < 6 yrs old and involves the deep spaces of the pharynx. Usually the result of extension of another infection.

Peritonsillar Abscess
Spread of bacterial tonsillitis into deeper tissues, causing an abscess

Epiglottitis
Infection of the epiglottis, which has become rare in children since the *H. influenzae* vaccine

P

Pharyngitis
Group B Strep: Treat with penicillin or macrolide. Consider steroids in cases with considerable swelling.
Chlamydia/Gonorrhea: Macrolide plus fluoroquinolone. Partners must be treated.
Most pts can be discharged home if tolerating oral intake.

Retropharyngeal Abscess
Admit for IV antibiotics and possible surgical drainage.
Consult ENT or oral and maxillofacial surgery for surgical evaluation.

Peritonsillar Abscess
Can be drained in the ED with needle aspiration.
Consider discharge home if pt is able to tolerate oral intake and take oral medications.
Antibiotics should include anaerobic coverage (e.g., penicillin and/or clindamycin).

Epiglottitis
Do not agitate the child, and be prepared to intubate and/or perform surgical airway if child loses airway. Consult ENT and anesthesia for possible elective intubation in the OR.
Adults typically need a period of observation in the ICU to ensure that the airway remains patent.
Start antibiotics and steroids.

Toothache/Fractured Tooth — HEENT

S **What are the pt's current symptoms?**
If the pt has pain, did it start gradually or abruptly? Is the pain localized to one tooth or multiple teeth?
- Upper dental pain may be secondary to sinusitis and is typically gradual onset with multiple teeth involved.

Has the pt had any dental work done recently?
"Dry Socket" or alveolar osteitis can occur 2 to 4 days after a dental extraction, and it is caused by the alveolar bone being exposed to air and getting inflamed.

If pt had a traumatic avulsion of the tooth
When was the tooth knocked out?
- After 1 hr, the chance of reimplantation is extremely low.

If a child, is the tooth a primary or secondary tooth?
- Never reimplant a primary tooth because it can affect the development and eruption of permanent teeth.

How has the pt attempted to preserve the tooth?
- Ideally, the tooth should be stored in saliva or "Hanks solution." If the pt wiped the tooth off, there is an extremely good chance that the periodontal ligament was wiped off, and reimplantation will not be successful.

Does the pt know where all of the teeth are?
- If multiple teeth were lost and the location of them is unknown, there is a chance that they were forced up in to the maxilla/mandible or swallowed.

If pt fractured a tooth, does he or she have the piece that is missing?
Ensure that the particle was not swallowed or aspirated.

Does the pt have any allergies?
If pt is allergic to novacaine (an ester), typically can be anesthetized with lidocaine/bupivacaine (amides) provided the lidocaine/bupivacaine are from single-use vials and do not contain a preservative. The preservative in lidocaine/bupivacaine is an ester and can cause an allergic reaction similar to novacaine.

Has the pt had any difficulty swallowing?
May signify a more serious deep-space infection. (See Pharyngitis p. 98.)

O **Perform a physical exam**
Evaluate all of the teeth and percuss for tenderness.
- Teeth are numbered with the #1 tooth being the upper right posterior molar (wisdom tooth) and extending across the mouth to the left upper posterior molar (#16). The #17 is the lower left posterior molar, and #32 is the lower right posterior molar.
- Instead of memorizing the tooth numbers, it is more important to know the names of the individual teeth (e.g., incisor (1), lateral incisor (1), canine (1), premolar (2), molar (3) per 1/4 mouth).
- Ellis classification is an ED terminology to describe the degree of fracture through a tooth. Dentists and oral and maxillofacial surgeons (OMFS) do not typically use the Ellis classification.
  - Ellis I: fracture through the enamel

- Ellis II: fracture extending into the dentin (creamy yellow color)
- Ellis III: fracture extending into the pulp (associated with bleeding)

Note any gingival tenderness or flocculence.
Ensure that there is no pharyngeal edema, erythema, or swelling.
Palpate maxillary sinuses to exclude sinusitis.

If unable to locate all missing teeth, consider obtaining the following x-rays

Panorex (panoramic x-ray) of maxilla and mandible that will demonstrate fractures and whether any tooth has been impacted into the jaw.
CXR: Ensure that a tooth was not aspirated. If seen in stomach, no intervention is required.

A

Toothache
From dental caries, fracture, alveolar osteitis, or periapical abscess
Typically will require a dental block in order to provide adequate pain control.

Tooth Fracture/Avulsion
If a permanent tooth has been avulsed for < 1 hr, an attempt at reimplantation should be made.

P

Toothache
Typically requires a dental block for adequate pain control.
Treat with antibiotics unless a periapical abscess is 100% excluded.
Arrange follow-up with dentist for definitive treatment.

Alveolar Osteitis
Irrigate socket with normal saline and pack with eugenol gauze.
Advise pt to keep the area moist.

Tooth Avulsion
Dental or OMFS consult is typically needed if your department cannot splint the tooth.
Irrigate the socket and ensure that there is no blood clot in the base.
Reimplant tooth and splint to teeth on either side.
Arrange follow-up with dentist in 2 to 3 days.

Tooth Fracture
Provide adequate anesthesia.
Refer Ellis III fractures to dentist ASAP.
Ellis I fractures can be treated by filing down the sharp edges and referral to a cosmetic dentist.
Ellis II fractures should be covered with dental cement and referred to dentist in the a.m.

VII
Genitourinary

Acute Renal Failure

S — What are the pt's current symptoms?
Common symptoms include:
- Nausea/vomiting
- Oliguria or anuria
- Hematuria
- Abdominal pain
- Edema
- Lethargy
- Shortness of breath

Has the pt had decreased oral intake or excess fluid losses?
Dehydration caused by decreased intake, diarrhea/vomiting, or excessive insensible losses can progress to prerenal azotemia and renal failure.

Has the pt had any recent infection or sore throat?
Increases suspicion for poststreptococcal glomerulonephritis.

What medical problems does the pt have?
Diabetes, hypertension, congestive heart failure (CHF), and connective tissue disorders (e.g., vasculitis) can all contribute to renal failure.

Cirrhosis can lead to renal failure as a result of third spacing and intravascular depletion (prerenal renal failure) or from loss of autoregulation from failure to clear cytokines (hepatorenal syndrome).

What medications does the pt take?
ACE-inhibitor and NSAID use can inhibit the kidney's autoregulation of blood flow and lead to renal failure.

Diuretic use with excessive fluid loss can cause renal failure.

Recent IV contrast administration and antibiotics (e.g., aminoglycosides) can cause acute tubular necrosis (ATN).

Has the pt had any surgical procedures or interventions done recently?
Vascular surgery, cardiac catheterization, or angiograms can lead to cholesterol embolization and secondary renal failure. Typically occurs 1 to 2 wks after the procedure.

Obtain a social history
Intravenous drug abuse increases the risk for embolic disease because of impurities in the drug or endocarditis, both of which can lead to acute renal failure.

Tobacco use increases the risk of atherosclerosis.

O — Evaluate the pt's vital signs
Perform orthostatic vital signs to exclude postural hypotension and dehydration.

Perform a physical exam
Lungs: Rales? Wheezing? Look for signs of volume overload and CHF.
Cardiac: Note any murmurs or S3/S4. Murmurs may suggest endocarditis; S3/S4 is seen with CHF. Note any pedal edema.
Abdomen: Ascites? Costovertebral angle tenderness? Peritoneal signs? May suggest infection.
Neurologic: Mental status changes? Caused by uremia, infection, or dehydration.
Skin: Any rashes to suggest strep infection?

Obtain the following labs
CBC: Evaluate for anemia, which may be the cause of renal failure or a result of it. Increased WBC can be seen with infection.

BUN/Creatinine: Usually elevated. BUN/Creatinine ratio > 20 suggests prerenal cause.

Electrolytes: Hypo-/hyperkalemia can be seen with renal failure. Ensure that calcium, phosphorus, and magnesium are normal.

LFT: Exclude liver disease.
Urinalysis: May see proteinuria, hematuria. Casts seen with intrinsic renal disease. May see eosinophilia with cholesterol emboli.
FeNa: Fractional excretion of urine sodium. If FeNa < 1, renal failure is typically because of prerenal causes.
Consider serum serologies if vasculitis or rheumatologic cause is suspected.
Obtain blood cultures if postinfectious or if endocarditis is suspected.

Obtain an ECG
Exclude cardiac ischemia and secondary CHF as cause.
Exclude hyperkalemic ECG changes that can quickly progress to cardiac arrest.

Obtain a CXR
Evaluate heart size and whether there is any pulmonary edema to suggest CHF.

Consider renal ultrasound
Evaluate renal parenchyma and exclude postrenal causes (e.g., obstruction).

Evaluate postvoid residual
Useful to exclude an obstructive or postrenal cause of renal failure.

A ### Acute Renal Failure
A rapid decline in renal function over hour to days
Causes are divided into prerenal, renal, and postrenal.
Prerenal causes are generally from low intravascular volume or low cardiac output.
Renal causes include ATN, vasculitis, glomerulonephritis, cholesterol emboli, etc.
Postrenal causes are from an obstruction in urine outflow and result in renal damage by increasing tubular pressures.

Differential Diagnosis
- CHF   - Anemia   - Cirrhosis

P ### Treatment is aimed at treating the underlying cause of the renal failure
All pts should have a Foley catheter placed to obtain accurate measurement of urine production.

Consider emergent dialysis in any pt who has
Significant acidosis
Hyperkalemia that is not responding to conservative treatment or pt who has ECG changes
Fluid overload with respiratory compromise

Stop any nephrotoxic agent
If prerenal disease is suspected, aggressively hydrate the pt
Disposition
Admit all pts. Mortality from acute renal failure is approximately 50%.
Consult Nephrology.

S — What are the pt's current symptoms?
Common symptoms include:
- Scrotal pain
- Dysuria
- Fever
- Tenderness to testicle/epididymis

May also complain of:
- Penile discharge
- Scrotal swelling
- Abdominal pain

Was the onset of pain gradual or abrupt?
Pain caused by epididymitis tends to be gradual in onset (> 24 hrs) and may involve both testicles.

What helps alleviate the pain? What increases the pain?
Epididymal pain typically increases when the pt stands and is relieved with scrotal support or by lying down.

Does the pt have a history of an STD?
Epididymitis in the young (20 to 30 yrs old) is associated with chlamydia and gonorrhea infections.
Common not to have any urethral discharge at time of presentation.

Has the pt been struck in the groin/testicle?
Exclude trauma from infectious etiologies.

Has the pt had a recent viral infection?
Orchitis is commonly associated with viral infections (e.g., mumps, coxsackie A).

Does the pt have any history of urinary retention or recent instrumentation of urinary system?
Epididymitis in older men is associated with *E. coli*, *Klebsiella*, or *Pseudomonas* and is commonly associated with urinary retention or recent instrumentation.

Obtain a PMH/social history
Include a sexual history and history of STDs.
Inquire specifically about benign prostatic hypertrophy because it increases the risk of urinary retention.

O — Evaluate pt's vital signs
Fever is more commonly associated with a viral syndrome.

Perform a physical exam
Abdomen: Tenderness? Peritoneal signs? Costovertebral angle tenderness?
- Exclude other pathology.

GU: Penile discharge? Scrotal swelling? Epididymal tenderness or swelling? Testicle swelling? May all be seen with infection. Inguinal hernia? May suggest incarceration. Cremasteric reflex? If absent, suspect testicular torsion.
- *Prehn's sign*: Decreased pain when testicles and scrotum are lifted; seen with epididymitis, but pain should not change with testicular torsion.

Rectal: Prostate tenderness or fullness? Suggests prostatitis.

Obtain the following labs
Urinalysis: May see WBC with epididymitis.
Urethral swab for gonorrhea/chlamydia: Exclude STDs.
Consider sending HIV and RPR if suspicion of STD-related epididymitis is high.
- Increased risk of HIV and syphilis if another STD is found.

If suspicious for testicular torsion, obtain scrotal ultrasound with Doppler flow
If there is any concern about testicular torsion, ultrasound should be obtained.

A ### Epididymitis
Inflammation or infection of the epididymis generally caused by retrograde spread of bacteria from the urethra or bladder.

Orchitis
Inflammation or infection of the testicle that can be caused by spread of infection from the epididymis or from hematogenous spread (e.g., viral).
50% of involved testicles will have residual atrophy.

Differential Diagnosis
- Hydrocele
- Testicular trauma
- Varicocele
- Renal colic
- Testicular torsion
- Inguinal hernia

P ### Provide effective pain relief
NSAIDs are generally effective.
Scrotal support with a jock strap.
Limit amount of standing/walking.

Start antibiotics
Sexually active males: Cover gonorrhea/chlamydia with fluoroquinolone (21-day course) or IM ceftriaxone plus doxycycline (10 days) or single-dose azithromycin.
Older males (> 35): Fluoroquinolone (21-day course)

Disposition
Most pts can be discharged home with follow-up with their primary care provider.
Admit pts who are unable to take oral medications or have evidence of an abscess that may require drainage.

S **What are the pt's current symptoms?**
Pain or swelling in the area of concern is the most common complaint.
Nausea/vomiting and fever can be seen with incarcerated hernias.

What was the pt doing when the swelling or bulge was first noticed?
An increase in the size of the hernia is normally associated with straining or lifting.

Does the pt have a history of a hernia or hernia repair?
Having a hernia on one side increases the risk of having a contralateral hernia.
Risk of hernia recurrence at the site of a former repair is 0.5% to 15%. Rate depends on location, type of repair, and co-morbid illnesses that may affect healing.

Is the swelling or bulge related to an area where surgery was performed?
Incision hernias typically appear 18 to 24 months after the surgery. Typically, pts will experience some dull pain in the area when they strain, and they will later notice the bulge.

Is the pt pregnant?
Femoral hernias commonly present in the 1st trimester of pregnancy.

Obtain a past medical history
Identify co-morbid illnesses.

O **Evaluate the pt's vital signs**
Perform a physical exam
Abdomen: While the pt is relaxed and lying supine, palpate the affected area for tenderness or mass.
- Palpate all incisions for defects in the fascia or mass.

GU: Place finger in external inguinal ring and have pt perform valsalva maneuver. With inguinal hernia, you can feel the hernia sac being pushed out through the ring.
- With large inguinal hernias, you may have abdominal contents in the scrotum, allowing one to hear bowel sounds in the scrotum.

Consider obtaining the following labs
Urinalysis: If you suspect urinary tract infection, pyelonephritis, or renal stone.
CBC: May show leukocytosis with strangulation.
Electrolytes, BUN, Creatinine: If pt is vomiting, to exclude electrolyte disturbance.

Consider obtaining a diagnostic study
Typically not necessary because diagnosis can be made with history and physical.
Abdominal x-rays can exclude obstruction.
Abdominal/Pelvic CT with oral contrast can show bowel loops or omentum in an abdominal wall defect.
Ultrasound/MRI can show abdominal wall defect and bowel.

A Hernia

Inguinal hernia: Can be direct (occur through Hasselbach's triangle) or indirect (occur through the internal inguinal ligament). Indirect hernias are the most common and are congenital, although they may not present until later in life.
Femoral hernia: Herniation into the femoral canal and are more common in women. Higher risk for incarceration and strangulation.
Incisional hernia: Occur at the site of a surgical incision.
Umbilical hernia: Occur because of a defect in the midline fascia. Higher risk of incarceration.

Differential Diagnosis
- Testicular torsion
- Bowel obstruction
- Epididymitis
- Lymphadenitis
- Hydrocele/Varicocele

P Asymptomatic hernias can be observed or repaired electively
Discharge pt home with instructions to return immediately for pain or if unable to reduce hernia.

Incarcerated hernias need to be reduced ASAP
The longer the hernia is incarcerated, the more edema will form in the bowel wall, making it harder to reduce.
- If the hernia has been incarcerated for more than 4 to 6 hrs, the pt will require surgical intervention to reduce the hernia and remove any necrotic bowel. Do not attempt to reduce.

To reduce the hernia, have the pt lie supine and relax.
- Provide analgesia and sedation as needed.
- Place constant, gentle pressure over the mass (herniation) until you are able to push it into the abdominal cavity. Pt should have immediate pain relief.

The definitive treatment for all hernias is surgical correction
Reducible hernias can be repaired electively.
Pts with evidence of bowel obstruction, nonreducible hernia, fever, peritonitis, or intractable pain should be admitted for urgent surgical correction.

S — What are the pt's current symptoms?
Most common symptom is painless swelling of the testicle.
- May have dull ache, but typically not painful.
- Pain typically only seen with large hydrocele/varicocele.

Pt may notice that the size of the testicle changes over time.
Hydroceles can be congenital in approximately 6% of males.
Varicoceles tend to occur in postpubertal males and are more common on the left.

Does anything increase the size or amount of tenderness?
Varicoceles tend to decrease in size when supine and increase in size with standing.
Hydroceles generally do not change with position and increase slowly over time.
- Exception is congenital hydroceles, which are generally communicating from a patent processus vaginalis and have direct flow of peritoneal fluid into the scrotal sac.

Is the swelling/pain unilateral or bilateral?
Bilateral varicoceles can occur in 33% of pts, but underlying testicular pathology needs to be excluded in lone right-sided varicoceles.
Congenital hydroceles are more likely to occur bilaterally.

Has there been any trauma?
Swelling may represent a hematoma.

Does the pt have any other medical problems?
Exclude other disease entities.

What medications has the pt tried?
NSAIDs may help reduce the size of hydroceles by decreasing the amount of fluid produced by the tunica vaginalis.

Obtain a review of symptoms
Fever and upper respiratory infection symptoms should your suspicion for viral orchitis/epididymitis.

O — Perform a physical exam
Abdomen: Tenderness? Masses? Peritoneal signs? Costovertebral angle tenderness? Exclude infection or alternative diagnosis.
GU: Penile discharge? Epididymal tenderness or mass? Inguinal hernia? Femoral hernia? Prehn's sign? Cremasteric reflex? Suggests alternative diagnosis. Testicular swelling or mass? Typically seen and tends to be nontender.
- Does the mass transilluminate? Darken the room and place a light source against the scrotum near the mass. The hemiscrotum should transilluminate if there is a hydrocele.
- Be sure to thoroughly exclude testicular torsion from your differential.

Obtain the following labs
Urinalysis: Typically normal. Done to exclude any infectious etiology.

Consider obtaining a scrotal ultrasound
If there is any concern at all about testicular torsion, a scrotal ultrasound with Doppler flow should be obtained.
Ultrasound can also help differentiate varicocele from hydrocele and may show any testicular compression with a varicocele.

A **Hydrocele**
An accumulation of fluid in the tunica vaginalis (the same layer that forms the peritoneal lining of the abdomen). Fluid can accumulate because of increased production or decreased absorption or can be caused by direct communication of the abdominal cavity with peritoneal fluid collecting in the scrotum. The latter is the common etiology in congenital hydroceles and may require surgical correction.
Acquired hydroceles are normally benign, although they can be a reaction to an underlying testicular pathology (e.g., cancer), which needs to be excluded if the hydrocele persists with conservative treatment.

Varicocele
Caused by dilation of the pampiniform plexus of spermatic veins. Occurs in the left hemiscrotum in most cases because of anatomic differences in venous drainage. It is rare to occur unilaterally on the right, and one-third of cases will be bilateral. Unilateral right varicoceles are rare enough that this finding must increase the concern for inferior vena cava obstruction.

Typically require surgical repair because they can lead to testicular atrophy and infertility.

P **Hydrocele**
Congenital hydroceles can be treated conservatively with observation, but they have a higher likelihood of needing surgical repair because they are more likely to communicate with the peritoneal cavity.
Supportive care consists of:
- NSAIDs
- Scrotal support
- Pt should follow up with primary care provider (PCP)/pediatrician/urologist to ensure improvement.

Varicocele
Supportive care if there is no evidence of testicular atrophy or if pt is done having children and is not concerned about fertility.
- Scrotal support
- NSAIDs
- Close follow-up with PCP/pediatrician/urologist to ensure that testicular atrophy does not occur.

Consult Urology for possible venous ligation of spermatic vein if there is evidence of retarded growth of the testis or testicular atrophy in young males.

Kidney Stones/Nephrolithiasis — Genitourinary

S

What are the pt's current symptoms?
Common symptoms include:
- Colicky, unilateral flank pain
- Nausea/vomiting
- Hematuria
- Dysuria

Does the pt's pain radiate anywhere?
Typically, the pain will radiate into the groin, penis, or testicles.

Does anything increase or decrease the pain?
Pain from nephrolithiasis tends to be abrupt in onset, colicky, and unchanged by any maneuvers or position changes.

Does the pt have any risk factors for kidney stones?
These include:
- Male gender
- Low water intake
- Immobilization
- High-protein diet (e.g., Atkin's)
- Family history
- Spinal cord injury
- Hypertension
- Malignancy
- Gout

Does the pt have a history of kidney stones?
Extremely common to have multiple recurrences of kidney stones.
Document whether the pt has undergone lithotripsy or surgical extraction of a stone in the past.

Has the pt had any fevers?
Not common with kidney stones alone, and a secondary infection will need to be excluded.

Has the pt recently been treated for a urinary tract infection?
Proteus and *Klebsiella* are associated with struvite stone formation because of their urea-splitting ability.

What medical problems does the pt have?
The following medical conditions are associated with increased kidney stone formation:
- HIV
- Cancer
- Gout
- Paralysis
- Primary hyperparathyroidism
- Renal tubular acidosis

Is the pt taking any medications?
Allopurinol and protease inhibitors are associated with kidney stone production.

O

Evaluate the pt's vital signs
Tachycardia and elevated blood pressure are common because of the associated pain. Note any fever that may signify an infection.

Perform a physical exam
General: Pts typically are unable to find a comfortable position.
Abdomen: Typically a normal exam. Pain is not reproducible.
- Note any costovertebral angle tenderness to suggest pyelonephritis.

Gyn: Exclude pelvic inflammatory disease (PID) and pregnancy.

Obtain the following labs
β-hCG: Necessary before x-rays are obtained and to exclude ectopic pregnancy.
BUN/Creatinine: Typically normal. May be elevated with complete obstruction.
Urinalysis: Microscopic hematuria seen in > 90% cases. Absence of hematuria does not exclude the diagnosis. Note any signs of infection (e.g., leukocyte esterase, WBCs).

Obtain a diagnostic study
Noncontrast helical abdominal CT scan: Gold standard. Will demonstrate stone, hydronephrosis from obstruction, and has the added benefit of being able to differentiate from an alternative diagnosis.
Renal ultrasound: Can exclude hydronephrosis from obstruction, but it is not sensitive enough to see all stones.
Intravenous pyelogram (IVP): Requires an IVP dye load and multiple radiographs. Not done routinely because of the amount of time it takes for the exam and dye load. CT scans are quicker and provide a lot more information.

A

Nephrolithiasis
There are four types of kidney stones: calcium oxalate/phosphate stones (80%), uric acid stones (10%), struvite stones, and cystine stones.
Knowing the type of stone can help direct treatment in order to prevent recurrences.

Differential Diagnosis
- Ectopic pregnancy   - Pyelonephritis   - PID
- Diverticulitis   - Appendicitis   - Ovarian cyst rupture

P

Provide effective pain relief
NSAIDs are very effective at alleviating the pain from kidney stones. IV/IM ketorolac can be used in pts with nausea and vomiting.
Narcotic pain medication may be needed initially.

Hydrate the pt with 2 L of normal saline
Treat nausea and vomiting with antiemetics
If stone is less than 5 mm in size
Most of these pts can be treated conservatively because the stone should pass on its own.
Educate the pt on the need to keep adequately hydrated and to drink plenty of liquids in order to flush the stone from the urinary tract.
- Pts should strain their urine so they will know when the stone is passed and can get it analyzed to see which of the four stone types it is.

Pain control should be provided with NSAIDs and narcotic pain meds.

Stones greater than 5 mm in size
Have a lower likelihood of passing on their own.
Discuss case with urologist. Pt may require lithotripsy, open pyelolithotomy, or percutaneous nephrolithotomy to remove the stone. Timing of intervention is generally based on the amount of obstruction seen on CT scan.

Antibiotics are generally indicated for any pt with fever or who has evidence of infection on urinalysis
IV ampicillin/gentamicin versus oral fluoroquinolone

Pyelonephritis/UTI

S
What are the pt's current symptoms?
Common symptoms include:
- Dysuria
- Urgency/Frequency
- Suprapubic tenderness/pain

In pyelonephritis, you may also see:
- Fever
- Nausea/vomiting
- Flank pain

Infants and elderly pts may only present with mental status changes, lethargy, or fever.

In males, has there been any penile discharge?
It is rare for males to get urinary tract infections (UTIs); the more common diagnosis is an STD.

In females, has there been any vaginal discharge or odor?
Vaginitis can cause dysuria.

Does the pt have risk factors for a complicated UTI or pyelonephritis?
These include:
- Pregnancy
- Recent antibiotic use
- Diabetes
- Immunosuppressed
- Neurogenic bladder
- History of self-catherization or indwelling catheter
- Recent hospitalization or residence in nursing home
- Recent instrumentation of urinary system

What medical problems does the pt have?
Multiple co-morbid illnesses increase the likelihood of admission versus outpatient treatment.

What medications is the pt taking?

Glucose, nitrite, blood, and bilirubin may be lower or falsely negative on urinalysis in pts who are taking vitamin C.

Obtain a social history
Inquire about sexual history and risk factors for STD/pelvic inflammatory disease (PID).

O
Evaluate the pt's vital signs
Perform a physical exam
Abdomen: Tenderness? May be seen with PID. Costovertebral angle tenderness? Seen with pyelonephritis.
GU: Inspect penis and testicles for tenderness and signs of STD.
Rectal: Prostate tenderness may be seen with prostatitis.
Gyn: Speculum and bimanual exam to exclude PID/vaginitis.

Obtain the following labs
Urinalysis: Elevated WBC, positive leukocyte esterase, and nitrite consistent with infection.
- Obtain clean-catch, midstream voiding specimen or straight cath urinalysis for most accurate results.
- Specimens with large numbers of epithelial cells suggests skin contamination.

Urine culture: Identify organism and antibiotic sensitivities.
CBC: WBC may be elevated with pyelonephritis.
β-hCG: Exclude pregnancy.

Consider sending blood cultures before starting antibiotics in pts with pyelonephritis who are going to be admitted.

Consider sending gonorrhea/chlamydia cultures in cases where you suspect an STD

Consider noncontrast helical abdominal CT or renal ultrasound if concerned about obstruction
Can show renal abscesses, stones, hydronephrosis, and obstruction.

A

Urinary Tract Infection
Infection of the lower urinary tract (cystitis)

Pyelonephritis
Infection of the upper urinary tract (kidney)

Differential Diagnosis
- Urethritis
- Cervicitis
- Prostatitis
- Vulvovaginitis
- PID
- Epididymitis

P

Consider phenazopyridine to provide some symptomatic relief of the dysuria
Inform pt that the phenazopyridine will discolor (orange) the urine, tears, and sweat and can permanently stain contact lenses and clothing.

Treat nausea/vomiting with antiemetics and provide IV hydration.

Start empiric antibiotics
Uncomplicated UTIs:
- Can be treated with 3 to 5 days of TMP-SMX or a fluoroquinolone.
- Other alternatives include nitrofurantoin or a cephalosporin.
- Pregnant pts are at high risk of developing pyelonephritis and should be treated with 10 days of cephalexin, nitrofurantoin, or amoxicillin.
- Children and pregnant women should not receive fluoroquinolones.

Complicated UTIs require treatment that will cover resistant organisms (e.g., *Pseudomonas*).
- 10 days of fluoroquinolone, aminoglycoside, or antipseudomonal cephalosporin

Uncomplicated (early) pyelonephritis:
- 10 to 14 days of fluoroquinolone, TMP-SMX, or oral third- or fourth-generation cephalosporin

Complicated pyelonephritis
- Fluoroquinolone, antipseudomonas penicillin/cephalosporin, and/or aminoglycoside

Discharge the following pts
Uncomplicated UTI
Complicated UTI and uncomplicated pyelonephritis provided the pt is able to tolerate oral medications and has close follow-up with primary care provider.

Admit pts
Requiring IV medications or who have complicated pyelonephritis

Consider urology evaluation
For anyone with multiple UTIs/pyelonephritis or any male over the age of 1 with a history of more than one UTI.

S — What are the pt's current symptoms?
Common symptoms include:
- Muscle pain or tenderness
- Nausea/vomiting
- Low-grade fever
- Dark brown urine

Has the pt done anything that may have caused the rhabdomyolysis?
Associated with overexertion (heavy lifting, exercise, or prolonged seizures), trauma (crush injuries), immobility (e.g., passed out on the floor for hours), and electrical/lightning injuries.

Has the pt recently been bitten by any animal or insect?
Brown recluse spider bites or snake bites can cause necrosis and secondary rhabdomyolysis.

What medical problems does the pt have?
Diabetic ketoacidosis, hyperthyroidism, seizure disorders, polymyositis, and dermatomyositis are all associated with rhabdomyolysis.
Inquire about any psychiatric disorders that may suggest neuroleptic malignant syndrome or serotonin syndrome.

What medications is the pt taking?
HMG-CoA reductase, zidovudine, and colchicines have all been associated with rhabdomyolysis or muscle injury.
Antipsychotics can cause neuroleptic malignant syndrome, which is characterized by high fever and rhabdomyolysis.

Obtain a social history
Cocaine, alcohol, and narcotic use can lead to muscle injury either from overexertion or prolonged immobilization while in a drug-induced coma.

Obtain a family history
Is there a history of any hereditary myopathies?

O — Evaluate the pt's vital signs
A markedly elevated temperature requires immediate attention and cooling measures to be initiated.

Perform a physical exam
Lungs, Cardiac: May note tachycardia.
Abdomen: Typically normal, but may have some mild tenderness.
Extremities: Note any muscle tenderness, stiffness, or rigidity.
- Ensure that there are strong pulses in all limbs.
- Consider compartment syndrome with any crush injury.
- Note any fractures.

Skin: Note any rash (dermatomyositis), bite marks, or areas of necrosis.

Obtain the following laboratory studies
CBC, Coags: Baseline measurements. Exclude anemia, infection, and disseminated intravascular coagulation.
BUN, Creatinine, Electrolytes: May have elevated BUN/Creatinine if there has been renal injury from rhabdomyolysis. Elevated phosphorus and potassium can be seen with cell lysis.
CK, CKMB: CK will be markedly elevated, but CKMB ratio should remain low.
- Degree of elevation correlates with degree of muscle injury.

Lactate dehydrogenase and uric acid: May be elevated.

Urinalysis: Macroscopic exam will be positive for blood, but microscopic exam will show minimum or no RBCs because of cross-reactivity of strip reagent with myoglobin in urine.

Obtain an ECG
Baseline and to confirm that there is no cardiac ischemia. Can see arrhythmias and ECG changes with electrolyte disturbances that occur with rhabdomyolysis.

Obtain x-rays of any suspected fracture sites
Check compartmental pressures if compartment syndrome is suspected

A

Rhabdomyolysis
Release of muscle's intracellular contents (creatinine kinase, potassium, calcium) from muscle injury and necrosis

It is extremely important to diagnose the inciting cause of the injury so that further injury can be prevented.

Differential Diagnosis
- Polymyositis/Dermatomyositis
- Acute renal failure
- Vasculitis
- Connective tissue disorders

P

Admit all pts
Will need frequent electrolyte monitoring and IV hydration.

Start aggressive IV hydration
Mainstay of therapy

Use normal saline.

Effective in facilitating clearance of myoglobin and preventing renal failure.

Goal for urine output is 200–300 cc/hr.

Once pt is intravascularly repleted, loop diuretics can be started to facilitate diuresis in addition to continuing the IV fluids.

Consider alkalinization of urine
Some authorities recommend bicarbonate infusion to help with clearance of myoglobin.

Need to monitor urine pH every 2 hrs. Goal for urine pH is > 6.5. Adjust bicarbonate infusion as needed to maintain this pH.

Monitor electrolytes every 2 to 4 hrs
Repeat as necessary and be prepared to treat hyperkalemia.

Treat inciting cause
Consider nephrology consult and dialysis
If pt has inadequate urine output and is developing signs of volume overload

S What are the pt's current symptoms?
Common symptoms include:
- Dysuria
- Polyuria
- Urethral discharge
- Conjunctivitis/uveitis
- Proctitis

Does the pt have a history of STDs?
Increased likelihood in individuals who have had a history of STDs.
May represent partial treatment, noncompliance with last treatment regimen, or reinfection.

Has there been any recent instrumentation of the urethral tract?
Symptoms may be caused by local inflammation from instrumentation.

What are the pt's risk factors for an STD?
Risk factors include:
- Multiple partners
- Inconsistent or nonexistent condom use
- New partners
- Partner with multiple other partners
- Alcohol or drug use

Does the pt have any rash or sores?
Painless chancre on penis or vagina is seen with syphilis.
Painful chancre can be seen with *Haemophilus ducreyi*.
Herpes has a classic rash consisting of vesicles on a base of erythema. "Dew on a rose petal."
Raised painless "bumps" or papules seen with condyloma acuminatum.

Is the pt pregnant?
Chlamydia has been associated with preterm labor and infertility.
Limits antibiotics that can be used to treat any infection.

Does the pt have any joint pain or arthritic complaints?
Reiter's syndrome (uveitis, urethritis, and arthritis) is associated with gonorrhea.

Obtain a thorough sexual history
Rectal intercourse or instrumentation should be asked about:
- Increases risk of HIV, Hepatitis B, Hepatitis C.

O Perform a physical exam
Male
- Penis: Inspect for penile discharge, rash, chancre, vesicles, or papules.
    - Be sure to retract foreskin if uncircumcised and return to normal position post-inspection.
- Testicles: Palpate for mass or tenderness.
- Rectal: Note any prostate tenderness.

Female
- Inspect for rash, chancre, vesicles, or papules.
- Perform speculum exam and note any cervical erythema or discharge.
- Perform bimanual exam and note any cervical motion tenderness, adnexal mass or tenderness, or uterine tenderness.

Obtain the following labs
Urethral or cervical swabs for chlamydia and gonorrhea.
Urinalysis to exclude urinary tract infection.
- In males, urinalysis should be obtained after urethral cultures so that any penile discharge is not flushed out.

HIV, RPR, Hepatitis B serologies to exclude co-infection.

A **Sexually Transmitted Disease**
Multiple infections typically coexist.
Ensure that all partners in the last 6 months are treated. Refer to local health department.
Become familiar with reporting requirements in your locale. Most states have mandatory reporting of all confirmed STDs.

P **General principles**
All pts should be educated on safe sex and birth control.
All partners will need testing and/or treatment.
Most pts should be treated empirically even if nothing is noted on physical exam.

Empiric treatment for chlamydia/gonococcal urethritis/cervicitis
Single-dose ceftriaxone, ciprofloxacin, cefixime, or ofloxacin plus single 1 g dose of azithromycin, or full course of erythromycin, doxycycline, or ofloxacin
Single 2 g dose of azithromycin can also be given, although it has a higher rate of side effects caused by GI upset.

Syphilis
Single dose of IM penicillin is effective in treating primary syphilis. Secondary and tertiary syphilis require longer treatment courses.
Doxycycline is recommended for individuals who are penicillin allergic.

Genital warts
Local treatment with cryotherapy or topical podophyllin.

Chancroid
Single dose of IM ceftriaxone or 1 g azithromycin is effective. A 3-day course of ciprofloxacin is also effective.

Genital Herpes
Oral antivirals, acyclovir, famciclovir, or valacyclovir for 7 to 10 days. Frequent recurrent outbreaks may require chronic suppressive therapy.

Testicular Torsion

Genitourinary

S | What are the pt's current symptoms?
Common symptoms include:
- Abrupt onset of testicular pain
- Nausea/Vomiting

Does anything alleviate the pain?
Typically, the pain is extremely intense and not relieved by any change in position or scrotal support.

How long has the pain been present?
Torsion of the testicular appendage is more common in children and typically presents as scrotal pain that has increased over several days.
Irreversible ischemic damage to the testicle from torsion occurs after 12 hrs.

Has there been any trauma or heavy physical exertion?
It is common for a testicular torsion to occur several hours after minor trauma or heavy exertion.
Nocturnal awakening with intense scrotal pain is common in children.

Has the pt ever experienced this pain before?
It is not uncommon for pts to have had intermittent testicular torsion in the past.

Has the pt had any dysuria, penile discharge, or hematuria?
Suggests alternative diagnoses (e.g., STD, kidney stone, urinary tract infection, epididymitis).

Obtain a medical history
A history of prior testicular torsion increases the risk for torsion on the contralateral side, if both testes were not surgically corrected.

Obtain a social history
Include a sexual history to ascertain risk of STDs.

O | Perform a physical exam
Abdomen: Tenderness? Masses? Peritoneal signs? Costovertebral angle tenderness? Suggests an alternative diagnosis, although may see tenderness.
GU: Penile discharge? Testicular swelling or mass? Epididymal tenderness or mass? Inguinal hernia? Femoral hernia? Prehn's sign? Tenderness and testicular swelling can be seen, but other signs suggest an alternative diagnosis.

- Check the cremasteric reflex: Assessed by stroking or gently pinching the skin of the upper thigh while observing the ipsilateral testis. The testis should elevate toward the perineum. The reflex is usually absent in pts with testicular torsion.
  - In order to get an accurate response, it is important that the pt be relaxed and that the room be warm.
- Testicular manipulation: If torsion is suspected, you can attempt to relieve the torsion by turning the testicle on its long axis away from the midline.
  - Success rate is generally low because testicle can be rotated 180 to 720 degrees.
  - Alleviation of pain is diagnostic of torsion.

Obtain the following labs
Urinalysis: Typically normal. Done to exclude any infectious etiology if diagnosis is unclear.

Genitourinary — Testicular Torsion

Obtain a scrotal ultrasound with Doppler flow
If diagnosis is clear based on history and physical exam, do not delay surgical evaluation and repair to obtain an ultrasound.
Color Doppler ultrasonography is the diagnostic test of choice to differentiate testicular torsion from torsion of the appendix testis or epididymitis.
- Hyperperfusion of the testis after detorsion can lead to an incorrect diagnosis of epididymitis.

A

Testicular Torsion
Congenitally absent or inadequate attachment of the testicle to the tunica vaginalis, which allows the testicle to twist on the spermatic cord, decreasing arterial blood flow.
Peak incidence in neonates and postpubertal boys.

Torsion of the Testicular Appendage
Leading cause of acute scrotal pain in children.
The testicular appendage is a small vestigial structure (remnant of the Müllerian duct system) on the anterosuperior aspect of the testis.

Differential Diagnosis
- Epididymitis
- Orchitis
- Hydrocele/Varicocele
- Kidney stone

P

Testicular Torsion
Obtain a Urology consult ASAP.
- Emergent surgical exploration and repair is needed to prevent testicular necrosis.
- Do NOT delay consultation to obtain laboratory studies or ultrasound.

Intermittent testicular torsion will need surgical repair, although it can be done on a more elective basis.
Provide pain relief with narcotics.
Disposition:
- Most pts will require admission or transfer for surgical exploration.

Torsion of the Testicular Appendage
Surgical removal of the appendage is not necessary, although it tends to increase the speed of recovery because pain can remain present with conservative treatment for weeks to months.
Conservative care includes:
- NSAIDs   - Scrotal support   - Ice to scrotum

Disposition:
- Most pts will be discharged home with follow-up arranged with primary care provider or urologist.

VIII
OB-GYN

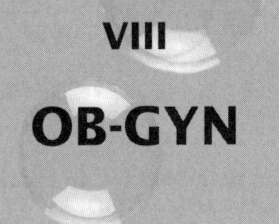

Ectopic Pregnancy

OB-GYN

S

Is the pt known to be pregnant?
Document pregnancy status and how pregnancy was determined (e.g., home pregnancy test, prior visit to physician).

When was the pt's last menses?
Determine the pt's due date and the current gestational age.
Ectopic pregnancies generally are diagnosed or rupture before 16 weeks gestation.

What symptoms is the pt currently having?
Common symptoms include:
- Vaginal bleeding
- Nausea/Vomiting
- Tachycardia
- Abdominal pain (may be mild)
- Syncope/Presyncope

Does the pt have any risk factors for an ectopic pregnancy?
- Pelvic inflammatory disease (PID)
- Intrauterine device use
- Prior ectopic pregnancy
- History of appendicitis
- Chemical ovulation induction
- Prior fallopian tube surgery
- Tobacco use
- Tubal ligation
- Endometriosis
- Prior abortion

Has the pt had an ultrasound done during this pregnancy?
Prior documented intrauterine pregnancy (IUP) essentially excludes diagnosis.

Obtain a complete Ob/Gyn history
Document number of pregnancies, miscarriages, abortions, and living children.
Document any history of STDs (e.g., Chlamydia, Gonorrhea).

Obtain a past medical history, medication list, allergy list, and social history
Inquire specifically about any prior abdominal surgeries.

O

Evaluate the pt's vital signs
Perform a physical exam
Abdomen: Note any tenderness and masses.
Gyn: Note any vaginal discharge or bleeding.
- Inspect cervix for discharge and bleeding. Note whether cervical os is open or closed.
- Palpate uterus for tenderness and masses. Note and estimate its size. An enlarged uterus does NOT exclude an ectopic pregnancy.
- Palpate adnexa for tenderness or masses.
- It is not unusual for the exam to be completely normal.

Perform rectal-vaginal exam to evaluate cul-de-sac for masses and stool for blood.
Complete the full physical exam.

Obtain the following labs
β-hCG: Obtain urine HCG to confirm pregnancy. If positive, obtain quantitative β-hCG.
Type and screen: Confirm Rh status in case anti-D imumunoglobulin needs to be administered.
CBC: Exclude anemia.
PT/PTT: If pt is unstable and may require surgery. Exclude a coagulation disorder.

Perform or obtain a pelvic ultrasound
Transvaginal ultrasound should show an IUP if β-hCG > 1500.

Transabdominal ultrasound should show an IUP if β-hCG > 5000.
Lack of IUP requires additional evaluation. Ultrasound may show an extrauterine mass and free fluid consistent with ectopic pregnancy.

If ultrasound is unavailable or nondiagnostic, consider performing a culdocentesis
Needle aspiration of fluid from the rectovaginal cul-de-sac. No consensus on a positive test, but generally 0.3 to 10 mL of unclotted blood is considered positive.

A **Ectopic Pregnancy**
Any pregnancy outside the uterus, with approximately 95% occurring in the fallopian tubes. Pain is thought to be caused by fallopian tube distention.
Second leading cause of maternal death, with an increasing incidence believed to be secondary to the increased incidence of PID.
Presentation is variable. A high degree of suspicion is needed in order not to miss any cases.

Differential Diagnosis
- Pregnancy
- PID
- Ovarian cyst
- Threatened miscarriage
- Inflammatory bowel disease
- Ovarian torsion
- Appendicitis
- Endometriosis

P **Provide supportive care**
Hemodynamically unstable pts should receive IV fluids and be cross-matched for blood products.
Administer anti-D immune globulin in any Rh-negative mother who has significant vaginal bleeding, is having a miscarriage, or has a documented ectopic pregnancy.

Obtain an Ob/Gyn consult ASAP for any pt who is unstable, has a documented ectopic pregnancy, or who is unlikely to follow up
Depending on age of gestation, an ectopic pregnancy can be treated medically with a methotrexate-induced abortion or surgical removal.
- Pts receiving methotrexate require serial β-hCG levels to ensure resolution of the pregnancy.

Disposition2
If pt is well appearing, hemodynamically stable, and the diagnosis is unclear, consider discharge home after consultation with Ob/Gyn.
- Arrange for serial β-hCG measurements. β-hCG should double every 2 days in a normal pregnancy and will decline in a miscarriage. A stable or slowly increasing level suggests an ectopic pregnancy.

Admit all pts who are hemodynamically unstable and/or will require surgical exploration.

S | What are the pt's current symptoms?
Typical symptoms include:
- Unilateral pelvic/abdominal pain that is typically sharp and sudden in onset seen with a ruptured ovarian cyst and torsion.
- Radiation of pain from groin to flank seen with ovarian torsion.
- Nausea/vomiting
- Fever

When was the pt's last menses?
Ruptured follicular cyst typically occurs at the time of ovulation, approximately 2 wks after last menses.
Ruptured corpus luteal cyst typically occurs just before menses.
Determine risk of current pregnancy.

Is there any vaginal discharge, vaginal bleeding, or fever?
Suggests a tubo-ovarian abscess (TOA) or pelvic inflammatory disease (PID).

Review the pt's past medical history
Document any prior STDs. Increases risk of TOA and PID.
Document any prior abdominal surgeries. Adhesions and scar tissue can increase the risk for ovarian torsion.

Review the pts Ob/Gyn history
Document any prior Ob/Gyn surgeries, STDs, PID, and pregnancies.

O | Evaluate the pt's vital signs
Ensure that pt is hemodynamically stable.

Perform a physical exam
Abdomen: Note any tenderness or peritoneal signs (e.g., rebound, guarding).
Gyn: Perform speculum exam and note any vaginal or cervical discharge/bleeding.
- Obtain Gonorrhea and Chlamydia cultures and wet prep.
- Perform a bimanual exam: Note any uterine tenderness or masses. Note any adnexal masses or tenderness.

Obtain the following labs
β-hCG: Exclude pregnancy and ectopic pregnancy.
Urinalysis: Exclude urinary tract infection (UTI)/pyelonephritis and hematuria seen with renal colic.
CBC: Exclude anemia. WBC may be increased in PID and TOA.

Obtain a diagnostic study
Pelvic ultrasound with Doppler: Study of choice. Doppler signal can demonstrate lack of blood flow to the ovary and diagnosis ovarian torsion. May also show TOA, ectopic pregnancy, pregnancy, and ovarian cysts. Free pelvic fluid can be seen with a ruptured ovarian cyst.
Abdominal/pelvic CT scan: Good sensitivity for TOA and free pelvic fluid. Less sensitive for ovarian cyst or ovarian torsion.

Ovarian Torsion/Cyst

A

Ovarian Torsion
Similar to testicular torsion. Twisting of the ovary on its vascular pedicle, causing ischemia and necrosis. Risk of occurrence increases with ovarian mass or venous congestion.

Ovarian Cyst
Pain can be caused by stretching of the capsule of the ovary or by rupture of the cyst and local peritonitis from blood or fluid.
Follicular cysts are small (∼2 cm) and occur midcycle, whereas corpus luteal cysts are large (up to ∼10 cm) and occur just before menses.

Tubo-Ovarian Abscess
An abscess of the ovary or fallopian tube that is typically associated with PID. Increased risk of infertility and ectopic pregnancy post-infection because of permanent scarring and damage to the fallopian tube.

Differential Diagnosis
- Appendicitis   - Ectopic pregnancy   - PID
- Endometriosis - UTI/Pyelonephritis - Renal Colic

P

Provide supportive care
Pain relief with NSAIDs and narcotics.
IV hydration if hypotensive.
Antiemetics for nausea/vomiting.

Consult Ob/Gyn ASAP for ovarian torsion and TOA
Pt may require exploratory laparotomy to diagnose and correct ovarian torsion.
TOA is typically managed with antibiotics, and pts undergo surgical drainage if peritoneal signs are present or pt does not respond to antibiotics.

Start broad-spectrum antibiotics with anaerobic coverage in TOA

Disposition
Admit all pts with TOA and those requiring surgery for ovarian torsion.
Pts with ovarian cysts who are hemodynamically stable can be discharged home with pain medications.

S   When was the first day of the last menstrual period?
Ensure that the last period was a typical period; if it was not normal for the pt, document the first day of the last normal menstrual period.
- Some women may have vaginal bleeding during their pregnancy that is similar to their menses, but it tends to be lighter and of shorter duration.

An accurate assessment of fetal age is extremely important in coordinating the pt's prenatal care.

Has the pt done any home pregnancy testing?
Current home pregnancy tests are extremely accurate, although false-negatives may be seen with dilute urine.

Is the pt having any symptoms consistent with pregnancy?
Common symptoms include:
- Amenorrhea
- Nausea (morning sickness)
- Breast enlargement/tenderness
- Increased urinary frequency

Obtain a complete Ob/Gyn history
Document prior pregnancies, miscarriages, and abortions.
Document any prior complications (e.g., gestational diabetes, preterm labor, premature rupture of membranes, miscarriages, still birth).
Document any history of STDs.

Document the pt's past medical history
Deep venous thrombosis/pulmonary embolism and miscarriages suggest antiphospholipid antibody syndrome and requires additional workup as an outpatient.

Review a medication list
Review the pregnancy classification of all medications the pt is taking and ensure that there are no class D or X medications.
If pt is on a class X medication, she should be counseled about the significant risk of birth defects.

Obtain a social history
Document tobacco, alcohol, or drug use.

O   Perform a physical exam
Obtain the following labs
β-hCG: Urine can detect levels > 25, serum > 10.
Urinalysis: Exclude urinary tract infection (UTI) if there are symptoms of polyuria.

Consider obtaining the following cultures
Gonorrhea, Chlamydia, and Wet prep if there is any history of STD disease, complaint of vaginal discharge, or vaginal bleeding.

A Pregnancy

Hyperemesis gravidarum: Nausea and vomiting that typically occurs in the 1st trimester and is associated with dehydration, ketonemia, and > 5% weight loss. Thought to be caused by elevated β-hCG levels as seen in multiple gestations or molar pregnancy.

Differential Diagnosis
- Gastroenteritis
- Ectopic pregnancy
- UTI
- Molar pregnancy

P Refer to Ob/Gyn for routine prenatal care

Early referral is recommended for high-risk pts (e.g., prior pregnancy complications) and if an accurate estimation of the fetal age cannot be made.

Determine the pt's estimated due date and current gestational age
Counsel pt on tobacco, alcohol, drug, and caffeine use
Refer pt to drug rehabilitation center if indicated.

Consider starting the pt on prenatal vitamins
Educate pt on morning sickness
Supportive care with small frequent meals, wrist bands, and antiemetics.

Counsel pt on her current medications
Discuss with primary care provider and/or Ob/Gyn stopping any class D or X medications and viable substitutes.
Discuss the risks of stopping medications abruptly.

Pelvic Inflammatory Disease

OB/GYN

S | What are the pt's current symptoms?
Common symptoms include:
- Vaginal discharge/odor
- Fever
- Vaginal bleeding
- Abdominal/pelvic pain
- Nausea/vomiting
- Dysparenia

Document the onset and duration of the pt's symptoms
Pain present > 3 wks is not likely to be caused by pelvic inflammatory disease (PID).

Does the pt have any risk factors for PID?
- Multiple sexual partners
- Age < 25
- History of STDs
- Use of intrauterine device
- Tubal ligation, strict condom use, and abstinence decrease risk for PID.

Document a complete Ob/Gyn history
Date of last menstrual period
Number of pregnancies, abortions, and miscarriages
History of STDs
Prior Gyn surgeries

Document past medical history, medication list, allergy list, and social history

O | Perform a physical exam
Abdomen: Note any tenderness or peritoneal signs (e.g., rebound tenderness).
Gyn: Perform a speculum exam. Note any vaginal or cervical discharge. Obtain Gonorrhea and Chlamydia cultures, wet prep, and KOH prep.
- Perform bimanual exam: Note any cervical motion tenderness, uterine tenderness or masses, or adnexal tenderness or masses.

Obtain the following labs
β-hCG: Exclude pregnancy and ectopic pregnancy.
Urinalysis: Exclude urinary tract infection (UTI)/pyelonephritis.
CBC: Leukocytosis may be seen.
ESR/CRP: Will be elevated.
- Consider sending RPR (to exclude syphilis) and HIV testing.

Consider obtaining a pelvic ultrasound to exclude an ectopic pregnancy or tubo-ovarian abscess if suspicious
May see free pelvic fluid with PID.

A — Pelvic Inflammatory Disease

PID is a clinical diagnosis. The presense of abdominal/pelvic pain, cervical motion tenderness, and adnexal tenderness meets CDC criteria for diagnosis.

An ascending infection of the female upper reproductive tract and the most common cause of pelvic pain in nonpregnant women.

PID is associated with an increased risk of infertility, ectopic pregnancy, and chronic pelvic pain.

Most cases are caused by *N. gonorrhea* and *Chlamydia trachomatis*.

Differential Diagnosis
- UTI/pyelonephritis
- Appendicitis
- Ovarian torsion
- Ectopic pregnancy
- Endometriosis
- Ovarian cyst

P — Provide supportive care

Treat pain with NSAIDs and narcotics as needed.
Treat nausea and vomiting with antiemetics.

Start antibiotic treatment

Requires a full 14-day course, not the single-dose regimen recommended for uncomplicated STDs.

Outpatient treatment regimens include:
- IM ceftriaxone (single dose) plus doxycycline 100 mg po bid for 14 days
- IV azithromycin (single dose) plus oral azithromycin 250 mg po daily for 7 days plus metronidazole 500 mg po bid for 14 days
- Fluoroquinolone plus metronidazole 500 mg po bid for 14 days

Counsel pt that all sexual partners in that last 3 months should be evaluated and treated

Disposition

Admit all pregnant pts and pts who appear toxic or are unable to tolerate oral medications secondary to nausea/vomiting.

Most pts can be discharged home and should follow up with their primary care provider or Ob/Gyn within 3 days.

S — Determine the who, what, when, and where of the assault

Attempt to interview the pt with a pt advocate, police, and physician in the room at the same time to minimize the emotional trauma to the pt.

The pt should remain fully clothed until after the interview is completed to minimize discomfort.

Document whether the pt has changed clothes, urinated, defecated, bathed, or douched since the incident.

Document whether a weapon or threat of harm was used.

Document the use of a condom and whether the assailant ejaculated.

Document the exact nature of the assault (e.g., fondling, intercourse, sodomy).

Did the pt suffer any injuries from the assault?
Document the exact location of all injuries and how they were obtained, if known.

When was the pt's last menses, and is the pt on any form of birth control?
Determine the need for pregnancy prophylaxis.

Determine the pt's past medical history, medication list, and allergy list
Obtain a social history
Document any recent alcohol or drug use.
Does the pt think she was drugged?

O — Perform a physical exam

Document any injuries. Obtain photographs, if possible.

Obtain evidence as directed by your local evidence collection kit. (Typically has paper bags to collect clothing, hair, nail clippings, and pubic hair, along with collection tubes for vaginal secretions and blood.)

Gyn: Perform a speculum and bimanual exam.
- Inspect for vaginal tears by using a toluidine swab, which turns tears blue.
- Obtain Gonorrhea and Chlamydia cultures.

Obtain the following labs
β-hCG: Exclude preexisting pregnancy.
HIV, RPR, Hepatitis B surface antigen and antibody: Baseline studies.
Consider sending a comprehensive drug screen if pt suspects she was drugged.

Obtain radiographs of any injuries where fracture is suspected

A **Sexual Assault**
Common, with 1 in 5 women being assaulted in their lifetime. Most do not report the crime. Men are also frequently victims of a sexual assault but rarely report it.

P **Provide supportive care**
Refer pt to a rape crisis center.
Consider psychiatric consultation if pt is very distraught or if there is evidence of posttraumatic stress disorder.
Treat traumatic injuries as needed.

Provide STD prophylaxis for Gonorrhea and Chlamydia
Single-dose regimen of ceftriaxone or fluoroquinolone plus azithromycin is ideal.

If pt is not immunized against Hepatitis B, consider administering Hepatitis B immune globulin in high-risk cases
Hepatitis B vaccination series should also be started.

Consider HIV prophylaxis treatment
Determining the HIV status of the assailant is often difficult.
HIV prophylaxis should be based on the type of assault (e.g., sodomy, intercourse, or fondling), local rate of HIV, status of the assailant if known, and the wishes of the pt after she has been appropriately counseled.

Consider pregnancy prophylaxis
Document a negative β-hCG.
Assault must have occurred within the last 72 hrs to be effective.
Standard regimen is ethinyl estradiol/norgestrel 2 tablets in the ED and two tablets 12 hrs later.
- Diphenhydramine can be administered 30 minutes before prophylaxis to help prevent nausea.
- Other regimens are equally effective.

Follow your local reporting guidelines for sexual assault
All states have mandatory reporting laws for sexual abuse.

Spontaneous Abortion ("Miscarriage")

S **Obtain a detailed history of the current complaint**
Document the first day of last menstrual period, current gestational age, and expected due date.
Quantify the amount of any vaginal bleeding present (e.g., pad or tampon count).
Document any abdominal pain or cramping to include time of onset, intensity, and any exacerbating or alleviating symptoms.
Verify the passage of any tissue (e.g., white matter/tissue) and whether the pt was able to save it for analysis.

Has the pt had a formal ultrasound with this pregnancy?
Confirm whether pt has single- or multiple-gestation pregnancy and presence of an intrauterine pregnancy.

Does the pt have any risk factors for miscarriage?
- Advanced maternal age (> 40)   - Alcohol/tobacco use   - Recent STD
- Increased gravidity (> 2)   - Prior miscarriage
- Caffeine > 100 mg/day   - Fever

Has there been any recent trauma or abuse?
Pregnant women are at increased risk for domestic violence.

Obtain a detailed Ob/Gyn history
Document prior pregnancies, miscarriages, or abortions.
Inquire about any complications with prior pregnancies.
Document any prior STDs/pelvic inflammatory disease.

Obtain a past medical history
Miscarriages, deep venous thrombosis, and pulmonary embolus have all been associated with antiphospholipid antibody syndrome.

O **Perform a physical exam**
Do not perform a pelvic exam in 2nd and 3rd trimester bleeding until after placenta previa is excluded by ultrasound.
Gyn: Perform speculum exam and note any vaginal or cervical discharge, blood in vagina, or blood coming from cervical os. Note any tissue in os or vagina. Document appearance of cervix (e.g., null parous, multiparous, open).
- Obtain Gonorrhea and Chlamydia cultures and wet prep.
- Perform a bimanual exam. Palpate the cervical os and note whether the inner os is open or closed.
Listen for fetal heart tones if > 12 weeks gestation.

Send the following labs
CBC, Coags: Exclude anemia and coagulopathy, and obtain a baseline in case there is heavy menstrual bleeding.
Quantitative β-hCG: Predicts ability to visualize fetus on ultrasound. Serial values will confirm spontaneous miscarriage.
Type and screen: Determine Rh status if unknown.

Obtain a pelvic ultrasound
Confirm intrauterine pregnancy. Document presence of fetal heart beat and position of placenta in 2nd and 3rd trimester pregnancies that present with bleeding to exclude placental previa.

A Spontaneous Abortion ("Miscarriage")
Most common complication of early pregnancy. Classified as:
- *Threatened abortion*: vaginal bleeding with closed cervical os
- *Inevitable abortion*: vaginal bleeding with open cervical os
- *Incomplete abortion*: vaginal bleeding with products of conception in vagina or cervical os
- *Complete abortion*: all products of conception expelled and cervical os reclosed
- *Septic abortion*: vaginal bleeding with fever, purulent discharge, and possible sepsis
- *Missed abortion*: in utero death of the fetus before 20 weeks with no expulsion of the products of conception

Vaginal bleeding in the 2nd and 3rd trimester
Placental abruption: placenta separates from uterus with formation of hematoma
Placenta previa: painless vaginal bleeding caused by placenta overlying the cervical os

Differential Diagnosis
- Ectopic pregnancy
- Molar pregnancy

P Provide supportive care
Resuscitate with IV fluids as needed.

Administer anti-D immune globulin in any Rh-negative pt
No surgical intervention is generally required for 1st-trimester miscarriages
Counsel the pt on typical course.
Arrange for serial β-hCG measurements to confirm diagnosis and ensure complete expulsion of products of conception.
Most pts will be discharged home.

Obtain an Ob/Gyn consult for any pt with 2nd and 3rd trimester bleeding
Admit pt.
Placental abruption requires emergent delivery.
Placenta previa with mild bleeding can typically be managed with observation.
- Emergent C-section is required for significant bleeding and fetal distress.

S Quantify the amount of bleeding
Can estimate bleeding by number of tampons/feminine hygiene pads used in a day.

Has the pt gone through menopause?
New onset of vaginal bleeding after menopause is worrisome for endometrial cancer.

Has there been any vaginal discharge, fever, abdominal pain, or nausea/vomiting?
Suggestive of an infection

Has there been any associated bruising, nosebleeds, rectal bleeding, or hematuria?
All are symptoms of a hypocoagulable state or disorder of platelet function.

Is the pt under increased emotional and/or physical distress?
Both can hinder normal ovulation and present with dysfunctional uterine bleeding (DUB).

Obtain a past medical history
Exclude secondary causes or co-morbid illnesses.
Polycystic ovarian syndrome, obesity, endocrine disorders (e.g., hypothyroidism, adrenal insufficiency) are all associated with disorders of menses.

Obtain an Ob/Gyn history
Document age of onset of menses, length of cycles, and typical duration of menses.
Document number of pregnancies and children (e.g., G1P1001).
Review current contraceptive use. Intrauterine devices associated with DUB.
Obtain a sexual history and document any history of STDs.

Obtain a medication list
Inquire specifically about contraceptive use, aspirin, and anticoagulants.

Document an allergy list, social history, and review of symptoms
Tobacco smoking has been attributed to DUB.

O Evaluate the pt's vital signs
Tachycardia and hypotension signify significant blood loss.

Perform a physical exam
Lungs, Cardiac, Abdomen: Typically normal. Abdominal tenderness suggests infection.
Gyn: Note amount of blood with/without clots in vagina. Note any vaginal discharge.
  Inspect for condyloma, lacerations, polyps, or foreign bodies as cause of the bleeding.
  - Obtain cervical cultures for gonorrhea and chlamydia.
  - *Uterus*: Note texture and presence of any masses to suggest fibroids. Tenderness suggests infection.
  - *Adnexa*: Note masses or tenderness.
Rectal: Palpate cul-de-sac for evidence of endometrial implants. Guaiac stool.

Obtain the following labs
Urine or serum β-HCG to exclude pregnancy.
CBC to exclude anemia and thrombocytopenia.
PT/PTT to exclude hypocoaguable state.
Gonorrhea/chlamydia cultures to exclude occult infection.
Type and screen if there is heavy blood loss and pt may need transfusion.

Consider obtaining the following labs
TSH if a review of symptoms suggests a thyroid disorder.
Prolactin to exclude prolactinoma.

Consider obtaining a pelvic ultrasound
Exclude ectopic pregnancy. Can demonstrate fibroids, thickened endometrium, and intrauterine blood with/without clots.

A

Dysfunctional Uterine Bleeding
Irregular bleeding caused by anovulation in the absence of organic disease.
Need to exclude other disorders before diagnosing the pt with DUB.

Menorrhagia
> 80 mL of blood loss or menses > 7 days in duration

Metrorrhagia
Vaginal bleeding not at the time of menses

Differential Diagnosis
- Pregnancy
- Endometriosis
- Endocrine disorder
- Infection
- Endometrial cancer
- Fibroids
- Coagulopathy
- Foreign body
- Anovulation

P

Provide supportive care
If hemodynamically unstable, administer IV fluids and consider blood transfusion.

Hormone Therapy
Minimal bleeding can be treated with 10 days of oral progesterone to stabilize the endometrial lining and then trigger a withdrawal bleed.
Moderate bleeding is best treated with oral contraceptives. Estrogen-only preparations control bleeding sooner.
Severe bleeding: IV estrogen or estrogen-only oral contraceptives followed by progesterone once bleeding is controlled.

Treat infections as identified
Refer pts with risk factors for endometrial cancer (e.g., hypertension, obesity, nulligravidas, long history of anovulation, diabetes, tamoxifen use or breast cancer) who are older than age 35 with new-onset bleeding to Ob/Gyn for endometrial biopsy

Disposition
Admit pts with severe blood loss who are hemodynamically unstable.
Most pts can be discharged home with follow-up arranged with primary care provider or Ob/Gyn.

Vulvovaginitis

S — What are the pt's current symptoms?
Common symptoms include:
- Vaginal discharge
- Pruritus
- Vaginal odor
- Dyspareunia
- May be asymptomatic and diagnosed on routine exam.

Obtain a detailed history of the current symptoms
- Duration of symptoms
- Any over-the-counter (OTC) treatment?
- Description of discharge
- Factors related to onset of symptoms

Inquire about actions/events that may have disrupted the normal vaginal environment
- Antibiotic use
- Antibacterial soaps
- Tampon/foreign body use
- Douching
- Change in sexual partner
- Increase in sexual intercourse

If symptoms are limited to the external genitalia, an allergic reaction is possible. Obtain an allergy review
New or improved detergents, soaps, lotions, or perfumes
New undergarments or clothing
Toilet paper or feminine hygiene products

Is the pt pregnant?
Pregnancy will limit treatment options, and infection may increase the risk of pregnancy complications.

Review the pt's past medical history, medication list, allergy list, and social history

O — Perform a physical exam
Gyn: Inspect labia for irritation, discharge, vesicles, edema, blisters, and erythema.
- Inspect vagina for foreign bodies, discharge, vesicles, excoriations, bleeding, or trauma.
- Check vaginal pH (normal 3.8–4.2).
  - pH > 4.5 consistent with bacterial vaginosis or trichomonas.
- Yeast infection: Cottage cheese–like discharge
- Bacterial vaginosis: Thin, dark, and homogenous discharge
- Trichomonas: Yellow-gray or green and frothy discharge
  - Inspect cervix for discharge, vesicles, or erythema.
  - Obtain wet prep, KOH prep, and gonorrhea and chlamydia cultures.
  - Complete pelvic exam and note any cervical motion tenderness, uterine masses or tenderness, or adnexal masses or tenderness.

Abdomen: Note any tenderness. Check for costovertebral angle tenderness.

Send the following labs
Wet prep: A drop of normal saline is added to a slide with a drop of vaginal discharge.
- Clue cells and WBCs seen with bacterial vaginosis.
- Trichomonads (mobile flagellated protozoa) and a large amount of WBCs makes diagnosis of *Trichomonas*.

KOH prep: A drop of KOH (10% potassium hydroxide) is added to a slide with a drop of vaginal discharge. KOH disrupts cell membranes except for fungal cell walls.
- Hyphae or pseudophyphae seen on prep makes diagnosis of *Candida*.

Gonorrhea/chlamydia cultures: Exclude coexisting infection.

Urinalysis: Exclude urinary tract infection. May need to obtain straight cath urine in order to prevent contamination from vaginal discharge.
Urine β-hCG: Document pregnancy status in all reproductive-age women.

A Vulvovaginitis

Bacterial vaginosis: Caused by overgrowth of *Gardnerella vaginalis* and is the most common cause of vaginitis. Associated with preterm labor, premature rupture of membranes, and endometriosis.

Trichomonas: Caused by protozoan, *Trichomonas vaginalis,* and is an STD. Also associated with preterm labor and premature rupture of membranes.

Candida vaginalis: Caused by overgrowth of yeast. *Candida albicans* being the most common. Second most common cause of vaginitis.

Differential Diagnosis
- Contact vulvovaginitis
- Cervicitis
- Genital herpes
- Atrophic vaginitis

P Bacterial vaginosis

Metronidazole or clindamycin are acceptable regimens. Avoid oral metronidazole in the 1st trimester of pregnancy.
- Metronidazole gel 0.75%, 5 g per vagina qd for 5 days
- Metronidazole 500 mg PO bid for 7 days
- Metronidazole 2 g PO in a single dose
- Clindamycin 2% vaginal cream 1 applicator qhs for 3 to 7 days

Trichomonas vaginitis
Treat pt and partner with metronidazole.
- Metronidazole 2 g PO in a single dose
- Metronidazole 500 mg PO bid for 7 days

Candida vaginalis
All medications are available OTC except for terconazole and fluconazole. Fluconazole should not be used in pregnant pts.
- Miconazole 2% cream 5 mg intravaginally for 7 days
- Terconazole 0.8% cream 5 g intravaginally for 3 days
- Clotrimazole 500 mg vaginal tablet for one dose
- Fluconazole 150 mg PO for one dose.

IX
Neurology

S — What are the pt's current symptoms?
Symptoms may range from mild memory loss to comatose state.
Common symptoms include:
- Mood swings
- Delusions
- Hallucinations
- Memory deficits
- Disorientation
- Psychomotor agitation

Was the change in mental status abrupt or gradual?
Abrupt onset can be a result of drugs, poisons, hypoglycemia, seizure, stroke, or trauma. Gradual onset can be a result of multi-infarct dementia, vitamin deficiencies, infection, Alzheimer's disease, drugs, or endocrine disorders.

Has the pt had any symptoms consistent with an infection?
In the young and elderly, it is not uncommon for the presenting symptom to be mental status changes with no other localizing complaints.

Has the pt been involved in any trauma or minor head injury?
Even relatively mild head injuries can result in subdural hematomas and mental status changes.

Does the pt have any other medical problems? Mental status changes can be seen with:
Hepatitis/Cirrhosis: Can lead to liver failure and hepatic encephalopathy.
Diabetes: Hypo- or hyperglycemia can progress to coma.
Chronic obstructive pulmonary disease/Asthma: Secondary to hypoxemia or hypercarbia.
Hypothyroidism/Adrenal insufficiency
Renal insufficiency: Secondary to uremia or decreased clearance of medications
Seizure disorder: Prolonged postictal state or status epilepticus.

What medications is the pt taking?
New medications, in particular narcotics, benzodiazepines, antibiotics, or herbal supplements, can affect your sensorium.
Chronic medications can also be implicated, especially if there has been any change in the pt's liver or renal function.

Obtain a social history
Is there any history of alcohol or drug abuse? Think of intoxication or overdose.
Any recent travel? Think about atypical infectious diseases.

Obtain a review of symptoms
Be thorough because it may be your only clue in determining the etiology of mental status changes.

O — Evaluate pt's vital signs
Consider rectal temperature (more sensitive than oral or tympanic).
Check SpO_2 and ensure that pt is not hypoxic.

Perform a physical exam
HEENT: Thyromegaly? Meningismus? Any signs of dehydration or head injury?
Lungs: Wheezing? Egophony? Are there any signs of respiratory distress or pneumonia?
Cardiac: Are there any signs of a myocardial infarction or congestive heart failure?
Abdomen: Peritoneal signs? Ascites? Any stigmata of liver disease?
Neurologic: Decorticate or decerebrate posturing? Weakness or numbness? Glasgow Coma Scale score?

Obtain the following labs
CBC: Leukocytes supports infection. Exclude anemia.
BUN/Creatinine, Electrolytes, LFT: Exclude renal, liver, and electrolyte disturbances.
Glucose: Exclude hypoglycemia.
Blood cultures: Exclude an occult infection.
Urinalysis, urine culture: Exclude urinary tract infection.
Urine drug screen, EtOH level: Exclude intoxication.

Consider lumbar puncture
If meningitis or encephalitis is suspected or no other cause is apparent

Consider ABG
Exclude hypoxemia, hypercarbia, or carbon monoxide poisoning.

Obtain an ECG
Exclude cardiac ischemia or arrhythmia.

Obtain a head CT
Exclude intracerebral bleed, epidural or subdural hematoma, or mass lesion.

Consider sending RPR, HIV, B_{12}, folate, ammonia level, aspirin, and acetaminophen
If history and physical suggests an infectious, metabolic, or toxic cause.

A ## Acute Mental Status Change
Treatment is aimed at correcting the underlying cause. The history and physical is essential in narrowing your differential.
Delirium: An acute, transient alteration in cognitive ability secondary to a physiologic event
Dementia: Chronic, irreversible change in memory and cognitive function

Differential Diagnosis
- Drug/alcohol intoxication
- Poison or toxic ingestion
- Uremia
- Hypoxemia/hypercarbia
- Hepatic encephalopathy
- Anemia

P ## Treat the underlying disorder
Start antibiotics for infections.
Stop offending medications.
Correct hypoxemia/hypercarbia.

Minimize sedation
Should only be used to prevent pts from hurting themselves or others.
Haldol and benzodiazepines either alone or in combination are effective.

Consider Neurology or Psychiatry consults as needed
All pts will need to be admitted
Admission to ICU, monitored bed, or regular bed should be based on pt's ability to protect the airway or anticipated progression of the disease process.

S   **Determine the PQRST of the pain.** (See Chest Pain p. 8.)
A sudden-onset "thunderclap" headache that is the worst headache of the person's life is the classic presentation of a subarachnoid hemorrhage.

Are there any associated symptoms with the headache?
Common for the pt to suffer from nausea/vomiting, photophobia, and phonophobia.
Sinus pain and pressure suggest a sinus headache.
Neck pain is common with tension or muscular headaches.
Complicated migraines may result in hemiplegia, ataxia, ophthalmoplegia, etc.

Did the pt experience an aura before the headache?
Auras can precede a migraine headache and include visual scotomas, paresthesias, aphasia, or the perception of a certain fragrance or taste.

Does the pt have a history of headaches?
Determine the frequency of the headaches and the typical severity.
Is this headache like all prior headaches?
Is there anything that causes the headache, or is it associated with a particular time of the month?
- Common for migraines to occur with a female's menses.

What has worked in the past to relieve the pt's headache?

Has the pt been exposed to any fumes or toxins?
Carbon monoxide poisoning or toxin ingestion can produce headaches.

Has the pt had any upper respiratory infection symptoms, fever, or neck pain?
Will need to exclude encephalitis/meningitis.

Does the pt have any other medical conditions?
HIV: Increases suspicion for atypical infection (e.g., toxoplasmosis) or mass lesion from Kaposi sarcoma.
Cancer: Consider brain metastasis.
Hypertension: Headache may be the first sign of hypertensive urgency/crisis.

What medications does the pt take?
Ask specifically about over-the-counter pain relievers because rebound headaches are common in those who take pain medication regularly.

Obtain a social history
In addition to alcohol, tobacco, and occupational histories, obtain a caffeine history. Withdrawal from caffeine can result in severe headaches.

O   **Evaluate the pt's vital signs**
Note any hypertension or fever.

Perform a physical exam
HEENT: Perform a fundoscopic exam. Sinus tenderness? Neck stiffness? Photophobia? Phonophobia?
Lungs, Cardiac, Abdomen: Typically normal.
Neurologic: Complete a full neurologic assessment. Exam is typically normal. May note paresthesias or hemiplegia.

Consider the following labs
ABG: Rule out hypoxemia, carbon monoxide poisoning, or hypercarbia.

ESR: May be elevated in temporal arteritis.
CBC: Exclude leukocytosis and anemia.

Consider obtaining a lumbar puncture
Exclude meningitis or encephalitis.
More sensitive than head CT in diagnosing a subarachnoid hemorrhage.

Consider obtaining a head CT
Should be obtained in any individual with neurologic symptoms, atypical headache features, new-onset severe "worst headache of my life" headache, or HIV with headache to exclude any underlying pathology.

A Headache
Common types of headaches include migraine, cluster, and tension headaches.
Migraine headaches are subdivided as migraine with or without aura or migraine variant.
- The exact etiology of migraines is unknown, but they are thought to be an imbalance of vascular regulation, resulting in vasoconstriction followed by vasodilation.

Cluster headaches are repetitive headaches that occur for weeks to months at a time, followed by periods of remission. Their exact etiology is unclear.

Tension headaches are the most common headaches seen and, although they were originally thought to be caused by muscle contractions, recent studies have shown that there is actually more muscle contraction with migraine headaches. The exact etiology of pain remains unclear.

Differential Diagnosis
- Stroke
- Meningitis
- Temporomandibular joint syndrome
- Carbon monoxide exposure
- Brain metastasis
- Temporal arteritis
- Sinusitis
- Subarachnoid hemorrhage

P Provide effective pain relief
Oxygen: Very effective in aborting the pain associated with cluster headaches.
Antiemetics: Prochlorperazine and metoclopramide are very effective in relieving headaches in addition to the nausea associated with them. Low abuse potential. Risk of extrapyramidal side effects.
Analgesics: NSAIDs, narcotics, acetaminophen, caffeine. Increased risk for withdrawal headaches and narcotic dependence.
Ergotamine: Causes vasoconstriction. Risk of coronary ischemia or hypertension.
Tryptans: Serotonin agonists that cause vasoconstriction. Same risks as ergotamine.

Consider starting prophylactic treatment if headaches are frequent, debilitating for several days, or extreme in intensity
β-blockers, SSRIs, calcium channel blockers, valproic acid, and tricyclic antidepressants have all been shown to decrease the frequency and severity of headaches.

Disposition
Most pts can be discharged home.

Meningitis

S
What are the pt's current symptoms?
Common symptoms include:
- Fever
- Nausea/vomiting
- Headache
- Mental status changes
- Neck stiffness
- Photophobia

Does the pt belong to a high-risk group?
- Elderly
- HIV positive
- College student
- Neonates
- Post-splenectomy
- Recent neurosurgical procedure
- Alcoholics
- Immunosuppressed

Has the pt been on antibiotics recently?
Antibiotics will make it more difficult to interpret the results of any cerebrospinal fluid (CSF) studies.

Has the pt been vaccinated against *N. meningitides*, *H. influenzae*, or *S. pneumonia*?
Vaccines do not completely prevent infection.

> *N. meningitides* vaccine only protects against serotypes A, C, Y, or W-135.

Has there been any trauma or recent head injury?
Supportive of an alternative diagnosis (e.g., subarachnoid or intracerebral hemorrhage).

Has the pt been exposed to anyone with meningitis?
Bacterial meningitis is only spread through close personal contact (live in the same household or spend prolonged time in an enclosed space with the index case).

Has the pt suffered any insect bites recently?
Increased incidence of aseptic (viral) meningitis in the summer, with mosquitoes being a common vector.

What other medical problems does the pt have?
Cancer (metastatic spread of tumor to meninges) and autoimmune disorders are associated with aseptic meningitis.

What medications is the pt taking?
Meningeal symptoms can occur from chemical or drug reactions.

Obtain a social history
Inquire specifically about living situation, close personal contacts, and any recent travel. Alcohol and drug use increase the risk for meningitis.

O
Evaluate the pt's vital signs
A fever does not need to be present.

Perform a physical exam
HEENT: Sinus tenderness? (Nasopharyngeal area is the most common source of infections.) Rhinorrhea? Dental abscess? Neck stiffness? Perform a fundoscopic exam to exclude papillary edema (may need to dilate eye to get adequate exam).

- *Brudzinski sign*: Reflexive hip and knee flexion when the neck of the supine pt is passively flexed.

Lungs, Cardiac, Abdomen: Typically normal. Note any signs of pneumonia or endocarditis as possible source of infection.

Extremities: Petechiae may be seen with *N. meningitides*.

- *Kernig's sign*: Neck and hamstring pain when the supine pt with hip and knee flexed at 90 degrees as the knee is passively extended.

Neurologic: Mental status changes? Weakness? Numbness?

Obtain the following labs
CBC: May see leukocytosis.
Blood cultures: Isolate causative organism.
Urinalysis, urine culture: Exclude urinary system as source of infection.

Perform a lumbar puncture
Head CT scan is only required before lumbar puncture if there is a risk of a mass lesion or elevated intracranial pressure.
Send fluid for cell count, glucose, protein, and Gram stain/culture.
- Consider sending fungal or tuberculosis cultures, latex agglutination studies, herpes simplex virus (HSV) polymerase chain reaction.

A Meningitis
Bacterial: *S. pneumoniae, N. meningitides,* or *H. influenzae* are the most common causes. Classic CSF findings are WBC > 1000, decreased CSF to serum glucose ratio, increased protein (> 150), and elevated opening pressure.
Viral: Classic CSF findings are WBC < 1000, normal glucose, protein > 200.
Autoimmune, chemical, and carcinomatous tend to have viral CSF picture.
Elderly and newborn pts require a high index of suspicion because they tend to have atypical presentations.

Differential Diagnosis
- Migraine
- Stroke
- Brain abscess
- Intracerebral hemorrhage
- Mass lesion

P Start empiric antibiotic treatment ASAP
Do not withhold antibiotics because there will be a delay in obtaining a CT scan or lumbar puncture.
Typical empiric regimen consists of 3rd-generation cephalosporin plus vancomycin (covers cephalosporin-resistant *S. pneumoniae*) $\pm$ acyclovir (if HSV is suspected).
Consider adding ampicillin to cover *Listeria* in the elderly, immunosuppressed, or neonatal pt.

Withhold any medications that may be related to a chemical meningitis
NSAIDS, sulfa, OKT3, COX-2 inhibitors, pyridium, and azathioprine

Place the pt in respiratory isolation
Consider starting steroids in children
Decreases risk of residual hearing deficits.
Ideally, the steroids should be given before the antibiotics.

Disposition
Admit all pts to an isolation room.
Contact your health department or infectious disease department if you suspect bacterial meningitis so that close contacts can be tracked down and given prophylaxis with ciprofloxacin or rifampin.

Seizures

S Was the seizure witnessed?
Unless tonic-clonic activity was witnessed, pt may have had a syncopal episode instead of a seizure.
- Small muscle twitches can be seen with syncope.

Does the pt have a history of seizures? If pt has known seizures:
Document last known seizure and typical frequency of seizures.
Why was the pt transported to the ED for this seizure?
- Bystanders called 911 before pt being able to inform them that this is the norm.
    - Atypical seizure?   - Prolonged seizure or postictal state
    - Injured?
- Has there been any change in the pt's medications?
    - Missed dose   - Increased/decreased dose   - New medication
- Does the pt experience an aura before seizures?
    ◆ May experience visual, gustatory, or olfactory changes.
- What type of seizure does the pt typically have?
    ◆ *Generalized seizure*: loss of consciousness with or without tonic-clonic activity
    ◆ *Partial seizure*: localized seizure that does not have to result in loss of consciousness, although may have impaired mentation

Is this a new (first) seizure?
Need to exclude secondary causes of seizure. These include:
- Head injury   - Drug reaction   - Metabolic disturbances
- Stroke   - Intracerebral bleed or mass   - Infection
- Alcohol or benzodiazepine withdrawal

Is the pt pregnant?
May be presenting symptom of eclampsia.

What medical problems does the pt have?
May suggest secondary causes of new-onset seizure.

What medications is the pt taking?
Numerous medications and herbal supplements can lower the seizure threshold and cause iatrogenic seizures.

Obtain a social history
Detailed alcohol and drug abuse history is required. Alcohol or drug intoxication/withdrawal have been attributed to seizures.

Obtain a review of symptoms
Exclude other causes of unconsciousness (e.g., syncope, hypoglycemia, sleep disorder).

O Perform a physical exam
Postseizure exam is typically normal.
Exclude any injury.
Pt may be postictal as exhibited by confusion, agitation, or a prolonged state of unconsciousness.
- If unconscious, ensure that pt is not in status epilepticus.

Obtain the following labs
CBC: Exclude infection, anemia, thrombocytopenia.
Electrolytes, Glucose, BUN/Creatinine: Exclude electrolyte disturbances, hypoglycemia, uremia.

Seizures

Drug levels: Ensure that pt's medications are therapeutic.
Consider sending the following labs:
- Prolactin: Elevated in true seizure, normal in pseudoseizure.
- Urine Drug Screen/EtOH level: Exclude intoxication.
- Urinalysis, ESR: Exclude infection.

Consider obtaining a head CT
Should be obtained if there is a change in the seizure pattern or characteristic, head injury, fever, or if this is a new-onset seizure.

Consider obtaining an electroencephalogram STAT if there is concern about status epilepticus

A

Seizure
A change in normal behavior caused by brain dysfunction
Status epilepticus: Seizure lasting > 30 minutes or recurrent seizure without a return to baseline.
Two classification systems:
- Primary vs. secondary (no apparent cause vs. known cause)
- Generalized vs. partial

Differential Diagnosis
- Syncope
- Narcolepsy
- Meningitis
- Migraines
- Hypoglycemia
- Pseudoseizure

P

Provide supportive care
Maintain airway.
Provide supplemental oxygen.
Establish IV access.

Treat underlying disorder if resulting from secondary causes
If pt is actively seizing, treat with
Benzodiazepines, phenytoin, or phenobarbital
Goal is to get pt's seizures under control in < 30 minutes to prevent permanent brain injury.

If drug levels are subtherapeutic, consider giving an additional dose
Disposition
Known epileptics can typically be discharged home if their mental status returns to normal and they have appropriate follow-up arranged.
Consult Neurology on all pts with new-onset seizures, persistent mental status changes, or focal neurologic deficits.
Consult local ordinances concerning requirements to report individuals having seizures to the department of motor vehicles.

Stroke

S **What are the pt's symptoms?**
Symptoms are variable. Common symptoms include:
- Expressive or receptive aphasia
- Mental status changes
- Nausea/vomiting
- Weakness/hemiplegia
- Impaired vision
- Ataxia

How long ago did the symptoms start?
If exact onset of symptoms can be determined to be less than 3 hrs, pt may be a candidate for thrombolytics.
- Difficult to ascertain when pt awakens with deficits or is found with them.

Have the symptoms resolved?
Transient ischemic attack (TIA) is defined as a transient neurologic deficit that resolves within 24 hrs, although most resolve within 5 minutes.

Has the pt had a stroke before? Are the current symptoms an exacerbation of past deficits?
Sleep deprivation, infections, and electrolyte disturbances can exacerbate prior deficits.

Does the pt have any risk factors for a stroke?
Risk factors include:
- Atherosclerosis
- Atrial fibrillation
- Hypertension
- Diabetes
- Smoking
- Amphetamine/cocaine use

What medical problems does the pt have?
Identify risk factors and co-morbid illnesses.

What medications is the pt taking?
Warfarin use increases the risk for hemorrhagic stroke.

O **Perform a physical exam**
HEENT: Nystagmus suggests cerebellar infarct. Palpate carotid arteries and listen for carotid bruits (diminished pulse or bruit suggests decreased blood flow).
Lungs, Cardiac, Abdomen: Typically normal. Irregular heartbeat may be heard with atrial fibrillation. Murmur may suggest endocarditis.
Extremities: Typically normal.
Neurologic: Evaluate mental status, speech, and short- and long-term memory. Measure strength in all four extremities. Evaluate cranial nerves. Check reflexes, tone of muscles, and Babinski reflex.

Obtain the following labs
CBC, electroytes, BUN/creatinine, glucose, coagulation studies, urinalysis: Exclude other causes of weakness or mental status changes.
Consider urine drug screen in young pts who may have used cocaine/amphetamines.

Obtain a noncontrast head CT
Done to exclude hemorrhagic infarct.
Typically normal. May see hypodense (dark) area in subacute strokes.

Consider MRI of brain
More sensitive for ischemia. Can show ischemic infarcts acutely.

Consider lumbar puncture if suspicious of subarachnoid hemorrhage
Head CT and brain MRI can miss small subarachnoid hemorrhages.

Stroke

A | **Cerebral Vascular Accident**
Caused by abrupt, focal interruption of blood flow to the brain
May be hemorrhagic (15%) or ischemic.
Ischemic infarcts can occur from embolisms, thrombosis, arterial stenosis, arterial dissection, or venous occlusion.

Differential Diagnosis
- Seizure
- Hypertensive encephalopathy
- Hypoglycemia
- Encephalitis
- Meningitis
- Drug effect

P | **Provide supportive care**
Maintain airway.
Provide supplemental oxygen.
Obtain IV access.

Consider thrombolytics
In moderate to severe ischemic strokes less than 3 hours in duration
Consider transfer to a stroke treatment center.

For ischemic strokes
Start the pt on aspirin.
Heparin may increase the risk of hemorrhagic complications, and no studies have shown a clear benefit to its use. Discuss starting it with the pt's primary care provider or neurologist.
Monitor blood pressure, but do not treat hypertension unless it exceeds 220/115.
- Hypertension may be protective and the brain's attempt to autoregulate blood flow. Decreasing the blood pressure may extend the infarction into watershed areas.

For hemorrhagic strokes
Consult Neurosurgery to consider surgical intervention.
Correct any coagulopathy or thrombocytopenia ASAP.

Disposition
All pts with neurologic deficits need to be admitted to the ICU or Neuro floor, where they can receive frequent neurologic checks.
Pts with TIAs that return to baseline quickly can be discharged home, provided that they are started on antiplatelet therapy and have close follow-up arranged for outpatient evaluation of the TIA.

S | What are the pt's current symptoms?
Common symptoms include:
- Peripheral vertigo
  - Nausea/vomiting
  - Tinnitus
- Central vertigo
  - Intact hearing
  - Vision changes
  - Ataxia
- Increased symptoms with head movement
- Fatigable nystagmus
- No change with head movement
- Nonfatigable nystagmus

Is the pt complaining of dizziness?
Dizziness is a nonspecific complaint. Have pt clarify whether he/she means vertigo (room spinning) or lightheadedness (near syncope).

Does the pt have or recently had any upper respiratory infection symptoms?
Peripheral vertigo (e.g., labyrinthitis) is associated with viral infections.

Are the symptoms abrupt in onset and intermittent or have they gradually progressed?
Peripheral vertigo is associated with a more acute onset and intermittent symptoms, whereas central vertigo tends to be gradual in onset and more persistent.

Quantify the severity of the symptoms, duration, and whether any inciting event or activity brings the symptoms on
What has the pt done to help improve symptoms?
Helpful to narrow differential and determine what an effective treatment might be.

What medical problems does the pt have?
Central vertigo can be associated with mass lesions, migraines, strokes, multiple sclerosis, peripheral vascular disease, and intracerebral hemorrhages.
Peripheral vertigo can be seen with acoustic neuromas, meningiomas, and post-trauma.

What medication is or has the pt been on recently?
Numerous medications have ototoxicity (e.g., aminoglycosides, loop diuretics, chemotherapeutic agents). A thorough medication history is needed.

Obtain a social history
Exclude drug or alcohol abuse as etiology.

O | Perform a physical exam
HEENT: Note any nystagmus (vertical, horizontal, or rotary) and whether it is fatigable. Evaluate tympanic membranes to exclude otitis media.

- Perform Dix-Hallpike maneuver: Have the pt sit on the bed, turn head to one side, and then lay supine quickly so the head can hang off the end of the bed. Note any nystagmus (type and duration). Raise pt to a seated position rapidly and note any nystagmus. Repeat with the head turned to the opposite side.
- In peripheral vertigo, this maneuver should exacerbate symptoms and show nystagmus that is short in duration (< 1 minute), fatigable, and starts after a short latency period.
- Central vertigo will last > 1 minute, has no latency period, and will not be fatigable. Symptoms are generally mild.

Lungs, Cardiac, Abdomen: Typically normal.
Neurologic: Complete a full neurologic exam to exclude any deficits that would suggest a central cause.

Labs are generally not helpful
Obtain to exclude secondary causes if suspected.

Obtain a noncontrast head CT
If pt has central vertigo, focal neurologic deficits, or any evidence of trauma or stroke

Consider obtaining an MRI
Increased sensitivity for cerebellar disease and early cerebrovascular accident (CVA).

A

Vertigo
Central Vertigo: Caused by brainstem or cerebellar disease. Common etiologies include CVA, intracerebral hemorrhage, cancer (metastatic or primary central nervous system), multiple sclerosis, or migraines.
Peripheral Vertigo: Most common is benign positional vertigo, which occurs from crystal forming in the semicircular canals. Dix-Hallpike maneuver may be diagnostic and therapeutic.
- Other causes include labyrinthitis, acoustic neuroma, meningioma, and drug ototoxicity.

Differential Diagnosis
- CVA
- Seizure
- Migraine
- Syncope
- Hypoxia
- Drug intoxication

P

Pt with central vertigo should be admitted for a complete evaluation
Although symptoms may be mild, the causes are more ominous.

Peripheral vertigo care is supportive
Antiemetics for nausea and vomiting.
Antihistamines, scopolamine, and benzodiazepines have all been used as vestibular suppressants.

Perform Brandt-Daroff, Semont, or Epley maneuvers for benign positional vertigo
A series of head and neck movements that has approximately 60% success rate in alleviating symptoms. Goal is to move the canoliths in the semicircular canals into the utricle, where they cannot interfere with the function of the endolymph.
A modified Epley's maneuver can be taught for self-treatment at home.

Disposition
Admit all pts with central vertigo, intractable vomiting, or if diagnosis is unclear.
Discharge pts with peripheral vertigo who are able to tolerate oral intake, have a steady gait, and have close follow-up.
Consider ENT consult for pts with persistent or severe symptoms.

S

Has the weakness been gradual in onset or abrupt?
Abrupt onset is more typical of cerebrovascular accident (CVA).
Gradual onset seen with multiple sclerosis (MS), amyotrophic lateral sclerosis (ALS) (Lou Gehrig's disease), myasthenia gravis (MG), Eaton-Lambert syndrome (ELS), and myopathies.

Does the pt have true muscle weakness?
Functional weakness (pt feels weak but there is no loss of muscle strength) can be caused by medical conditions such as exercise intolerance, joint pain, anemia, congestive heart failure, or depression.

Does the weakness improve with exertion?
ELS tends to improve with exertion, whereas MG gets worse.

Does the pt have any visual complaints (e.g., diplopia, blurred vision)?
MS, ELS, and MG typically have visual complaints. ALS has normal vision and sensation.

Does the pt have any muscle pain or tenderness?
Suggests dermatomyositis or polymyositis.

Does the pt complain of any alteration in sensation (e.g., paresthesias)?
ALS and MG do not affect sensory functions.

What activities is the pt having difficulty doing?
Proximal muscle weakness is characterized by an inability to rise from a seated position associated with deltoid, quadriceps, and axial muscle group weakness.
Distal muscle weakness is characterized by decreased grip strength, foot drop, and wrist flexion/extension. Pt may have difficultly opening jars and standing on tips of toes.

What medical problems does the pt have?
MG is associated with autoimmune disorders (e.g., autoimmune hypothyroidism, rheumatoid arthritis, systemic lupus erythematosus).
70% of ELS pts will have a cancer (most common small cell lung cancer), but the neurologic symptoms often develop before the cancer is diagnosed.
Dermatomyositis and polymyositis also have an increased incidence in cancer pts.

What medications is the pt taking?
Chronic steroids, antimalarial agents (e.g., chloroquine), penicillamine, and colchicine have all been attributed to muscle weakness.

Obtain a social history and a review of symptoms
Living in the northern latitudes before puberty increases the risk for MS.

O

Perform a physical exam
HEENT: Perform a fundoscopic exam to look for optic neuritis. Note nystagmus, weakness of extraocular movement, ability to swallow.
Lungs, Cardiac, Abdomen: Ensure adequate respiratory effort and strength.
Extremities: Check for muscle atrophy, tenderness, or rash.
Neurologic: Perform a complete exam to include functional testing (e.g., open a jar, stand from seated position). Rate strength of all major muscle groups. Check reflexes in all limbs and Babinski signs.

Obtain the following labs
CBC: Exclude anemia.
Electrolytes: Exclude hypo-/hyperkalemia, hypo-/hypercalcemia, and hypomagnesemia.
CK: Elevated in myositis and myopathies.
Blood cultures, urinalysis, and urine culture: Exclude occult infection.
TSH: Exclude hypothyroidism.

Consider obtaining a head CT
Exclude intracranial hemorrhage and CVA.

Consider obtaining a chest CT
Evaluate for enlarged thymus (MG) and lung cancer.

A Weakness
Multiple sclerosis: Most common autoimmune inflammatory demyelinating disease of the central nervous system. Onset is 20 to 40 years of age.
Amyotrophic lateral sclerosis: Most common motor neuron disease characterized by upper and lower motor neuron degeneration.
Myasthenia gravis: Autoimmune disease characterized by the development of acetylcholine receptor antibodies.
Eaton-Lambert syndrome: Paraneoplastic autoimmune disease similar to MG with a high association with small cell lung cancer.

Differential Diagnosis
- Botulism   - Tick paralysis   - Guillain-Barré syndrome
- Stroke   - CNS tumor   - Hypothyroidism

P Consider a Neurology consultation
Provide supportive care: IV hydration, supplemental oxygen

Disposition
Admit all pts with new onset of symptoms who do not have a diagnosis.
- Monitor respiratory status closely because progressive respiratory muscle weakness may require intubation. Follow forced vital capacity and negative inspiratory pressure.

Pts with known disease, mild symptoms, and no signs of respiratory compromise can be discharged home if close neurologic (same or next-day) follow-up is arranged.

Treat any underlying electrolyte disturbance or infection
Inpatient testing to be considered
MRI of brain: More sensitive for demyelination and inflammation associated with MS.
Lumbar puncture: Exclude occult infection. Oligoclonal bands and elevated IgG seen in MS.
Muscle biopsy: Denervation seen with ALS. Inflammation seen with myositis.
Electromyogram: To differentiate muscle from nerve abnormalities.
Acetylcholine receptor antibody: Positive in 85% of MG pts.
Tensilon test: Edrophonium challenge will temporarily reverse symptoms in MG pts.

X
Trauma

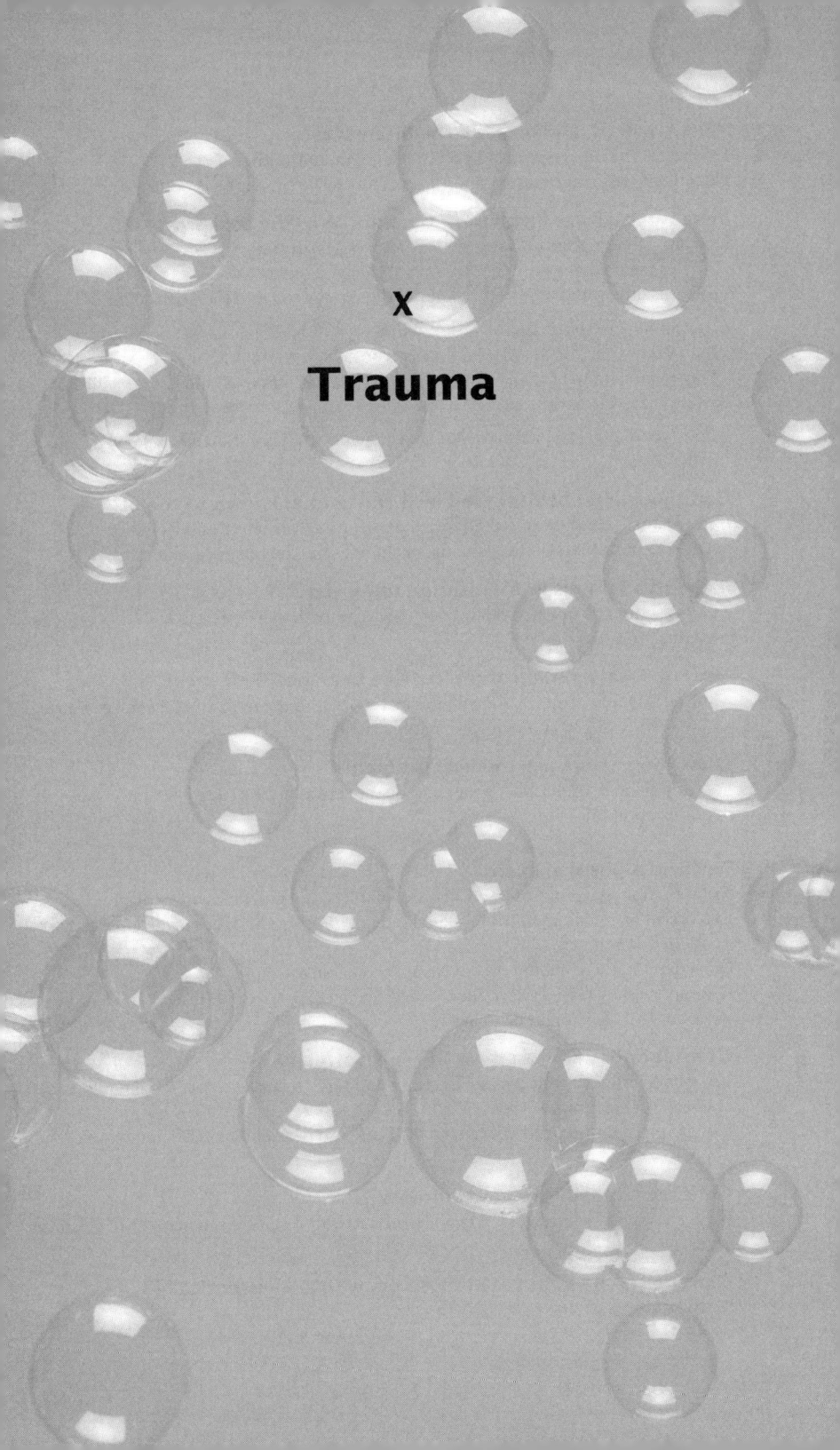

Animal Bite

S

When, where, and how did the bite occur?
Document the time, place, and events leading up to the bite.
Document the areas of injury and whether any self-treatment has occurred.

What animal was involved in the bite? Was the bite provoked?
Dog bites are usually associated with a crush or tearing injury.
Cat bites are typically puncture wounds and have a higher associated risk of osteomyelitis with the introduction of bacteria directly into the periosteum.
Wild animal bites increase the risk of rabies exposure. Rodents (e.g., mice, rats, squirrels) except for the ground hog are considered a low risk for rabies transmission. There is no transplacental transmission of the virus, and most rodents are killed in the attack that would transmit the virus.
Unprovoked attacks or animals that are acting bizarrely are more likely to be infected with rabies.

Can the animal be observed or is the animal known to the pt?
If the animal cannot be observed for 10 days for signs of rabies and its rabies vaccination status is not known, the pt should start the rabies vaccine series.

Is the pt's tetanus immunization up-to-date?
Tetanus should be updated if last booster was more than 5 years ago and the wound is tetanus prone.

Has the local animal control service been notified?
Most jurisdictions require that all bites be reported to the local animal control warden. Check with your ED on reporting requirements.

Does the pt have any medical problems?
Pts with diabetes or peripheral vascular disease are at increased risk for infectious complications.

O

Perform a physical exam
Note location, size, number, and shape of all bites. Consider drawing a diagram.
Explore all wounds carefully to exclude foreign bodies, joint space involvement, or any bone/tendon injury.
Consider anesthetizing the area to ensure an adequate exam.
A complete skin exam is warranted, especially in children, to document any minor injuries that they might be unaware of.

Consider obtaining an x-ray of the involved area
Use x-rays judiciously to exclude fractures and foreign bodies. Most foreign bodies can be seen on plain films.
Ultrasound, fluoroscopy, CT scan, or MRI can also be useful in localizing foreign bodies.

Consider obtaining wound cultures
If the area appears infected or has purulence, a wound culture can help direct antibiotic therapy.

Consider blood cultures in those pts who are systemically ill appearing

Animal Bite

A Wound infections are common, involving 80% of cat bites and 5% of dog bites. Bacteria associated with infection include:
- Skin flora: *Staphylococcus* or *Streptococcus*
- Cats: *Pasteurella, Moraxella, Neisseria*
- Dogs: *Pasteurella, Capnocytophaga cynodegmi*

P **Wash wounds thoroughly and debride as needed**
Most wounds should be allowed to heal by secondary intention to minimize the risk of infection and abscess formation.
Consider primary closure of wounds on the scalp and face that can be disfiguring.

Ensure that tetanus immunization is current
Administer tetanus diphtheria vaccine if not current and pt has been immunized in the past.
If wound is tetanus prone and pt has not been immunized in the past, administer tetanus immune globulin and tetanus diphtheria vaccine.

Consider antibiotic therapy
Antibiotics should be prescribed for all distal extremity wounds and moderate- to high-risk wounds because of the high rate of infectious complications.
Amoxicillin/clavulanic acid is the antibiotic of choice. Clindamycin plus a fluoroquinolone or TMP-SMX is an alternative in penicillin-allergic pts.

Consult Orthopedics for any injuries that involve fractures, tendon involvement, or compromise the joint space
These wounds require extensive irrigation and debridement that is more suitable for the OR.

Consider rabies immunoprophylaxis
In high-risk wounds, pt should receive the rabies vaccine and rabies immune globulin. Treatment can be delayed if animal can be observed and is healthy appearing.

Disposition
Most pts can be discharged home on oral antibiotics.
Admit pts with systemic symptoms or joint infections, who fail to respond to outpatient therapy, or who have significant co-morbidities requiring IV antibiotics.

Ankle Sprain

S

How did the pt injure the ankle?
Document whether the pt inverted or everted the ankle.
Inversion injuries are associated with injury to the lateral malleolus and associated ligamentous structures.
Eversion injuries are associated with injury to the medial malleolus.

Has the pt been able to bear weight and walk since the injury?
Ask the pt how he or she got to the ED. Often, the triage nurse will place the pt in a wheelchair, but he or she was able to walk to the triage desk.
Inability to walk four steps is an indication to obtain x-rays.

Where does the pt localize the pain?
Localizes the area of injury and helps exclude foot injuries with referred pain.

What self-treatment has the pt done to date?
Pain medications and ice may alter your physical exam.

Document past medical history, medications, allergies, and social history
Exclude co-morbid illnesses, possible medication interactions with your prescribed treatment, and allergies.
Complete documentation is needed in order to bill.

O

Perform a physical exam
Note any tenderness, ecchymosis, or swelling.
- Specifically check for tenderness over:
  - Fifth metatarsal head: Exclude a Jones or dancer's fracture.
  - Navicular: Exclude fracture/dislocation.
  - Fibula head: Exclude a Maisonneuve fracture (proximal fibula fracture, disruption of the interosseous membrane, and medial malleolus fracture or deltoid tendon rupture).
Document normal sensation and pulses.

Perform the Thompson test
Ensure that the Achilles tendon is intact. With the foot in a neutral position, squeeze the calf muscles. Foot should plantar flex. Lack of movement suggests complete rupture of the Achilles tendon. Movement will be normal with partial ruptures.

Test the stability of the ankle joint
Anterior draw: Test the anterior talofibular ligament (ATFL). Push the tibia posterior while pulling the heel forward. Increased laxity or movement when compared to the unaffected side suggests injury.
Talar tilt: Tests ATFL and calcaneofibular ligament. Plantar flex the foot and test for laxity with inversion and eversion. Compare to the unaffected side.

Consider obtaining radiographs
According to the Ottawa ankle rules, an ankle series is indicated for:
- Inability to walk more than four steps
- Bony tenderness on posterior edge or tip of either malleolus
- Bony tenderness over 5th metatarsal head or navicular (include foot series)

Obtain a full tibia/fibula series if pt has pain over the proximal fibula.

A **Ankle Sprain**
Ligamentous sprain that is graded 1, 2, or 3:
- Type 1: mild stretch of the ligament with fibers remaining intact
- Type 2: partial disruption of ligament fibers
- Type 3: complete disruption of the ligament

ATFL is the most common tendon injured.

Achilles Rupture
Risk of rupture increased with use of prednisone, fluoroquinolones, and age older than 60.

Ankle Fracture
Foot Fractures
Jones fracture: Fracture of the 5th metatarsal.
Dancer's fracture: Avulsion fracture of the base of the 5th metatarsal.

P **Provide supportive care**
All injuries should be treated with Rest, Ice, Compression, and Elevation (RICE).
NSAIDs and narcotics may be needed for pain relief.

Ankle Sprains
Pt should bear weight as tolerated.
Severe (type 3) sprains should be treated with posterior splint, non-weight-bearing status, and referral to orthopedics.
Air or gel stirrup braces can help prevent recurrent sprains while allowing plantar and dorsiflexion.
Pts with persistent pain after 2 wks of conservative therapy should be referred to Orthopedics.

Achilles Rupture
Orthopedics consultation
Treatment is controversial. Options include operative repair or conservative therapy with casting and non-weight-bearing status.

Ankle Fractures
Orthopedics consultation for any open fracture or unstable fracture.
- Open fractures also require antibiotic treatment (i.e., cefazolin) and assurance that tetanus immunization is up-to-date.

Stable fractures can be managed with splint (posterior stirrup), non-weight-bearing status, and orthopedic referral.

Foot Fracture
Posterior splint
Orthopedics referral

Disposition
Most pts will be discharged home, with follow-up arranged with orthopedics or primary care provider.
Admit all pts with open or unstable fractures that will require operative repair.

S When, where, and how was the pt burned?
Document time and place of burn.
Document type of burn (e.g., electrical, thermal, or chemical).
- If chemical, attempt to identify exact chemical involved, and at a minimum, if it is an acid or alkali.
  - Acids cause coagulation necrosis, which limits depth of injury.
  - Alkalis cause liquefaction necrosis, resulting in deep penetration.

Systemic effects are possible.
Ask specifically what burned because toxic vapors can be released from the burning process.

What self-treatment has the pt tried?
Inquire about any ointments or creams that may have been applied because they can alter the burn's appearance, and depending on the cream/ointment, may increase the risk of infection.

Does the pt have any difficulty speaking or breathing?
Thermal burns of the airway and nasopharynx can result in dysphonia, and respiratory compromise from edema.
Bronchospasm, pneumonitis, and adult respiratory distress syndrome (ARDS) can all result from inhalation injuries.

Is the pt's tetanus immunization current?
All burns that involve the dermis are tetanus prone. Update if last booster was > 5 years.

Is the pt's or parent's story consistent with the injuries seen?
Consider child abuse in any child presenting with burns where the story does not match the pattern of injury seen.

Obtain a past medical history, medication list, allergy list, and social history
Sulfa allergy will prevent treatment with silver sulfadiazine.

O Evaluate the pt's vital signs
Monitor SpO_2 and ensure that oxygenation is adequate.

Perform a physical exam
Document location and thickness of burns.
1st-degree burn: superficial erythema (e.g., sunburn)
2nd-degree burn (partial-thickness): dermis involved; erythema, pain, and blistering present.
3rd-degree burn (full-thickness): painless; visible thrombosed vessels are pathognomonic.
4th-degree burn: full-thickness burn that includes muscle and bone
Body surface area of burns can be estimated by the rule of nines in adults.
- 9% of body surface area is given to each arm and head/neck.
- 18% for each leg, anterior torso, and posterior torso
- 1% perineum

Consult a Lund and Browder chart for estimating body surface area of burns in children.
HEENT: Note any soot or burns around nares and mouth. Note any singed nose or facial hair.
- Predicts upper airway injury and risk of respiratory compromise.

Lungs: Note any wheezing, consolidation, respiratory distress.
Cardiac, Abdomen: Typically normal. Tachycardia may be present.
Extremities: Ensure adequate range of motion if burns involve hands, or cross joints.

Consider obtaining the following labs
CBC, electrolytes, BUN, creatinine, ABG, carboxyhemoglobin: Exclude carbon monoxide poisoning, ensure proper oxygenation, and exclude electrolyte disturbance.

Obtain an ECG with any electrical injury
Exclude cardiac injury and arrhythmia.

Obtain a CXR if evidence of inhalation injury is present
Exclude pneumonitis, ARDS, underlying pulmonary disease.

A — Burn
Minor Burn: Involves < 15% of body (< 10% in elderly/children)
Moderate Burn: 15% to 25% of body (10% to 20% in elderly/children)
Severe Burn: > 25% (> 20% in elderly/children) or burns that may cause cosmetic or functional deficits (e.g., face, perineum, hands) or burns that compromise respiratory function

P — Ensure that pt has an adequate airway
Intubate for respiratory distress or if there are severe facial/neck burns. Early intubation is recommended because airway edema may preclude intubation later.

Provide IV hydration for moderate and severe burns
Burns require large fluid resuscitation. Use the Parkland formula to estimate fluid needs.

Ensure that pt's tetanus immunization is up-to-date
Booster required if last injection was > 5 years.

Oral and IV antibiotic prophylaxis are not needed for minor burns and are controversial in severe burns
Follow your local treatment protocols.

Local burn management
Dress minor burns with nonadherent dry gauze after applying topical antibacterial cream (e.g., silver sulfadiazine, Bactroban). Avoid using sulfadiazine on the face.

Provide effective pain relief
NSAIDs and/or narcotics for pain

Disposition
Follow local reporting guidelines if child abuse is suspected.
Consider transferring all severe burn pts to a local burn treatment center.
Minor burn pts can be discharged home with close follow-up.
Circumferential, electrical, moderate, and severe burn pts should be admitted.
2nd-, 3rd-, and 4th-degree burns may require skin and muscle grafts.

S — How, when, and where did the injury occur?
Attempt to identify the exact mechanism of injury. Helps predict the type of fracture.
Prolonged time to presentation for care, increases risk of compartment syndrome and rhabdomyolysis. Determine time of injury.
What treatment has the pt received before arrival in the ED?

Document pt's dominant hand
Plays an important role in deciding promptness of surgical repair or surgical versus conservative management of fractures.

Is it an open fracture?
Any fracture associated with an overlying laceration. An orthopedic emergency because of the increased risk of osteomyelitis if not cleaned and debrided early.
Document last tetanus immunization.

Does the pt have any weakness or numbness?
Exclude associated nerve injury.
Often pt will not want to move limb, but you must test strength and sensation distal to the fracture.

Does the pt have any other medical conditions?
Peripheral vascular disease, diabetes, and osteoporosis all may attribute to delayed bone healing and/or increased fracture risk.

O — Evaluate pt's vital signs
Tachycardia can be from pain but may also be the first sign of significant internal blood loss. A femur fracture can result in 1 L of blood loss.

Perform a physical exam
Fully expose any area of concern.
Document pt's ability to ambulate and any abnormality to the gait.
Note any tenderness, erythema, ecchymosis, deformity, crepitus, or decreased range of motion.
- On hip pain, document any leg-length discrepancy and position of leg when in position of comfort (e.g., internally or externally rotated).

Evaluate for ligamentous or tendon instability or tenderness.
Fully evaluate the joints above and below the area of concern.
Document sensation and strength before and after any movement or splinting of affected area.
Document pulse strength and quality along with capillary refill.
Complete a full exam to exclude any occult injuries.

Obtain x-rays of the concerned area
Ensure that x-ray includes the joint above and below the area of concern.
Need a minimum of two views (e.g., posteroanterior and lateral) to exclude fracture.
Describe the fracture:
- State whether it is open or closed.
- State the area of the fracture (e.g., epiphysis, metaphysis, diaphysis).
- State the type of fracture (e.g., transverse, oblique, spiral, greenstick, comminuted).
- State angulation, rotation, or displacement using the proximal fragment as your reference point.
- State any associated dislocation or joint involvement.

Consider obtaining the following labs if presentation is delayed
CBC, electrolytes, BUN, creatinine, creatinine kinase: Exclude rhabdomyolysis, secondary renal failure, and anemia.

A
Fracture
Can be caused by trauma, pathologic (e.g., metastatic bone lesions), or stress related. Open fractures require emergent orthopedic evaluation for aggressive irrigation and debridement in order to prevent osteomyelitis.

Differential Diagnosis
- Sprain
- Arthritis
- Contusion
- Tendon/ligament tear
- Dislocation

P
Provide effective pain relief
NSAIDs and/or narcotics are effective.
Rest, Ice, Compression, Elevation (RICE)

Open fractures
Irrigate with copious amounts of sterile normal saline.
Ensure that bone fragments remain covered with moist gauze soaked in normal saline.
Provide tetanus immunization if not current.
Administer IV antibiotics (e.g., cefazolin) as soon as possible.

Splint the affected area
Document neurovascular status pre- and post-splinting.
The splint should immobilize the joint above and below the fracture.

Disposition
Open fractures fractures/dislocations that cannot be adequately reduced, and fractures associated with neurologic deficits require immediate orthopedic referral.
Most hip or femur fractures are admitted for operative repair the following day.
All other pts can be discharged home after the fracture is splinted with Orthopedic follow-up.

S **How, when, and where did the pt get injured?**
If pt was assaulted, check to see what your local reporting requirements are.
Was the event witnessed? Attempt to get a first-hand account of the event.

Did the pt ever lose consciousness?
Document the time of unconsciousness and how the pt was after consciousness was regained.
- Was the pt confused? Can be seen with a postictal state resulting from seizure or closed head injury.
- Consider a syncopal episode if pt had loss of consciousness (LOC) for a few seconds and immediately awoke once he or she was lying down.

Pts who have an LOC, awaken, and have a *lucid period* and then develop a change in mental status or LOC likely have suffered an epidural hematoma (EDH).

Was any seizure activity noted?
Ask bystanders specifically what they saw because the layperson's idea of seizure activity varies.

Does the pt have a history of falls or head injuries?
Repeated falls or head injuries increase the risk of subdural hematomas (SDHs), especially in the elderly.

Does the pt have any neck pain?
Consider spinal injury in any pt who has a significant head injury.

Does the pt have any weakness, numbness, or paralysis now?
Indicates a more severe head injury with either a severe contusion or intracerebral bleed.

Does the pt have any other medical problems?
Document any prior head injuries or cranial surgery.
Cardiac history may suggest arrhythmia and secondary syncope.

What medications is the pt taking?
Inquire specifically about warfarin, aspirin, clopidogrel, and other blood thinners that can increase the risk of intracranial bleeding.

Obtain a social history
Document any recent alcohol or drug use. Both can obscure your evaluation of the pt's mental status.

O **Evaluate the pt's vital signs**
Glasgow Coma Score should be included as a vital sign.

Perform a physical exam
HEENT: Note any ecchymosis, lacerations, or abrasions.
- Inspect skull for any depressions or stepoffs consistent with fracture.
- Note any hematotympania or blood/cerebrospinal fluid (CSF) draining from ear.
- Inspect nares: Note bleeding or CSF drainage.
- Inspect mouth: Note any loose teeth, fractured teeth, or lacerations.
- Inspect neck: Note any vertebral tenderness or stepoff. Pt should be placed in a c-collar until x-rays are obtained, if there is any significant head injury.

Neurologic: Perform mental status exam. Test all cranial nerves. Note any focal weakness, numbness, Babinski's sign, or diminished or hyperactive reflexes.

Obtain a C-spine series
Exclude vertebral injury.

Obtain a head CT scan
Without contrast and with bone windows. Exclude skull fracture, intracerebral bleed, EDH, or SDH.
- Classic EDH appears as a convex hyperdensity with shift of midline structures, compression of ipsilateral lateral ventricle, and can lead to uncal herniation.
- Classic SDH appears as a crescent-shaped concave hyperdensity. Large SDH can also cause compression of the lateral ventricle.

Consider obtaining the following labs
CBC, coags, bleeding time: Exclude thrombocytopenia, hypocoaguable state, or platelet dysfunction if pt has significant bleeding or intracerebral bleeding.

Type and screen: If blood products (fresh frozen plasma or platelets) are needed to correct bleeding state.

EtOH level, urine drug screen: Exclude intoxication or drug effect as cause of mental status changes.

A Head Injury
EDH usually caused by a temporal-parietal skull fracture with laceration of the medial meningeal artery is the classic description. Death can result quickly from uncal herniation.

SDH usually caused by the tearing or laceration of bridging veins that transverse the subdural space. Associated with cerebral contusions, cerebral edema, and diffuse axonal injury.

Concussion: Diffuse reversible brain injury that occurs at the time of trauma. Characterized by a change in mental status with or without LOC (may last up to 6 hours).

Differential Diagnosis
- Seizure   - Syncope   - Cerebrovascular accident

P Supportive care
Ensure that pt is able to maintain airway, and intubate if needed.

Treat hypotension with normal saline. Hypertension should be treated very cautiously and typically does not require treatment.

Seizure prophylaxis with phenytoin is generally recommended.

Perform frequent neurologic checks.

Consult Neurosurgery for any epidural or subdural hematoma or intracerebral bleed
An EDH with impending herniation requires immediate surgical decompression. A burr hole may need to be placed in the pt's head in the ED as a temporizing measure.

Disposition
Pts with mild head injuries who have no neurologic deficits, a normal head CT scan, and have family/friends who can watch them closely can be discharged home.

Admit all pts with intracerebral bleeds, SDH, EDH, or neurologic deficits to the ICU for close monitoring and frequent neurologic checks.

Laceration

S **How, when, and where did the pt obtain the laceration?**
Primary wound closure (closure at time of initial evaluation) is generally not recommended if the laceration is more than 8 hrs old because of an increased risk of infection. Facial lacerations have been closed up to 24 hrs later in order to get a better cosmetic closure.
Lacerations caused by glass, wood, and other organic material have an increased risk for retained foreign bodies.
Abide by local regulations requiring reporting any child abuse or assault.
If wounds are suspicious for an assault, be sure to ask the pt how the lacerations were obtained in private because the companion may be the perpetrator.

Did the pt sustain a puncture wound to the foot?
Plantar puncture wounds have an increased risk of infection because of *Pseudomonas* and a retained foreign body if the pt was wearing shoes at the time.

When was the pt's last tetanus immunization?
If last immunization was > 5 years ago, pt will require a booster dose.

What other medical problems does the pt have?
Diabetes and peripheral vascular disease increase the risk for wound infections and delayed wound healing.

What medications is the pt taking?
Chronic steroid use will delay wound healing.

Document any medication allergies, social history, and review of symptoms

O **Evaluate the pt's vital signs**
Tachycardia is the first sign of significant blood loss. Hypotension is a late sign.

Perform a physical exam
Document the length, depth, shape, and location of all lacerations.
- Consider drawing a diagram.

Thoroughly irrigate and explore the wound to exclude underlying tendon, blood vessel, joint or muscular injury, and foreign bodies.
Document pt's handedness on all lacerations involving the arms or hands.
Evaluate the capillary refill, distal pulses, distal sensation, and the function of any underlying joints.
Complete a full physical exam to exclude any secondary injuries.

Consider obtaining an x-ray of the area involved

Plain radiographs can be invaluable in demonstrating foreign bodies. Glass (down to 2 mm in size with or without lead), gravel, and metallic bodies can easily be seen. Organic material (e.g., wood) and plastic are often missed.

Fluoroscopy, CT scan, or ultrasound can also be useful in localization of organic or plastic foreign bodies.

A **Laceration**
Differential Diagnosis
  - Bite   - Crush injury   - Open fracture

P Control bleeding
Apply direct pressure on the wound or just proximal to the wound.
A blood pressure cuff applied to the limb can be inflated to slow blood flow.
A local tourniquet can be applied to aid in controlling blood flow while the wound is being closed. Tourniquet time should be limited.

Provide pain relief
NSAIDs, narcotics, or local anesthetics can all be effective.

Update tetanus immunization
If wound is tetanus prone and pt has never received tetanus immunization, pt should receive tetanus immune globulin and a tetanus diphtheria vaccination.

Anesthetize the wound
Local or topical anesthetics can be used. Anesthetic with epinephrine can reduce the amount of anesthetic required and aid in controlling bleeding by causing vasoconstriction.
Consider a regional nerve block if local infiltration of anesthetic will alter wound edges and prevent a good cosmetic closure.

Irrigate the wound
The wound should be irrigated with a minimum of 500 cc normal saline (use more if heavily contaminated). A 30-cc syringe with an 18-gauge angiocatheter provides an ideal pressure stream to flush bacteria and debris without causing tissue damage.

Remove any foreign bodies that are visualized.

Debride the wound
Remove any devitalized tissue and revise the wound edges as needed to obtain a clean edge that will prompt wound healing.

Close the wound
Closure can be done with sutures, staples, topical skin adhesive, or skin-closure tape as indicated.
Ensuring that the wound edges are everted, there is minimum tension across the suture line, and the wound edges are lined up will provide for excellent cosmetic closure and prevent wound dehiscence.

Wound should be dressed with antibiotic ointment and dry sterile dressing. Consider splinting a finger or limb if the laceration crosses a joint

Disposition
Most pts will be discharged home to have their sutures or staples removed by their primary care provider.
General guidelines for suture/staple removal:
- Face: 3–5 days
- Scalp: 10–14 days
- Upper Extremity: 7–10 days
- Lower Extremity: 10–14 days
- Over Joints: 14 days

Admit pts with severe wound infections, joint involvement, or repairs that will require surgery.

Antibiotics are generally not indicated but should be given for bites, plantar puncture wounds, or heavily contaminated wounds

S **Determine the PQRST of the pain.** (See Chest Pain p. 8.)
Document if pain radiates, and particularly if it follows a dermatome distribution. Pts often present with back pain before a herpes zoster outbreak.
Pain radiating down the leg and past the knee is consistent with sciatica.

What exacerbates and alleviates the pain?
What movements, position, or activity increases the pain?
What has the pt done to help treat the pain? Does any activity or position decrease the pain?
Pain that is worse at night or with rest suggests a malignant or infectious cause.

Is the pain related to a traumatic injury?
Pain following a fall, motor vehicle crash, or direct blow requires x-ray evaluation to exclude fracture.

Has the pt had any bowel, bladder, or erectile dysfunction? Has the pt had any weakness or numbness?
Signifies a neurologic deficit and requires emergent evaluation and treatment.
Bowel, bladder, or erectile dysfunction is seen with cauda equina syndrome.
Weakness or numbness can be seen with a herniated disc and nerve impingement.

Has the pt had any fever or chills?
Will need to exclude an epidural abscess or osteomyelitis as cause of pain.

Does the pt have any other medical problems?
A history of cancer increases the risk for metastatic bone disease and fractures.
Osteoporosis increases the risk of spontaneous fractures.
A recent bacterial infection or recent back surgery/lumbar puncture increases the risk for epidural abscess.

What medications is the pt taking?
Chronic steroid use increases the risk for infection and osteoporosis with vertebral fractures.
Anticoagulation use increases the risk for a serious pathologic condition as cause of pain.

O **Evaluate the pt's vital signs**
Note any fever.
Tachycardia can be secondary to pain.

Perform a physical exam
Back: Palpate vertebrae and note any tenderness, deformity, or stepoff. Palpate the paraspinal muscles and note any tenderness or spasm.
- Evaluate the pt's gait and ability to bend forward, back, and laterally at the waist.
- Palpate the sciatic notch for tenderness.
- Perform straight leg raise (SLR): Pain that radiates below the knee is consistent with disc herniation. Should have pain when either leg is raised. SLR can be tested when leg is fully extended in seated position or when lying down.

Neurologic: Test strength in all muscle groups of the lower extremity. Evaluate sensation in all dermatomes. It is imperative that you have pt remove shoes and socks to test sensation of the foot. Evaluate deep tendon reflexes.

Rectal: Rectal tone and the bulbocavernous reflex should be evaluated in any pt who complains of bowel or bladder incontinence.

Obtain radiologic studies if indicated
Plain radiographs may show fracture, spondylitis, osteomyelitis, or spondylolisthesis.
CT scan offers increased sensitivity for bone fracture. CT myelogram can be done to exclude disc herniation in those unable to get an MRI.
MRI scan is the study of choice. Evaluates spinal cord, soft tissue, discs, and bone. An ideal exam to exclude disc herniation, epidural abscess, or spinal cord compression.

Consider obtaining the following labs
ESR: Typically elevated with osteomyelitis, epidural abscess, or metastatic disease.
CBC, blood cultures: May see elevated WBC count and identify causative organism.

A | Low Back Pain
Number-one cause of disability; 90% of population will experience back pain; and 2nd most common cause of physician visits.
10% of back pain is caused by a serious pathologic condition and 0.01% is caused by infection.

- Red flags include age < 20 or > 50, fever, history of cancer, immunosuppression, abnormal neurologic exam, pain increased at night or with rest, anticoagulation, and/or recent trauma.

Differential Diagnosis
- Arthritis
- Herpes zoster
- Referred abdominal pain
- Fracture
- Epidural abscess
- Degenerative joint disease/degenerative disc disease

P | Provide effective pain relief
NSAIDs, narcotics, acetaminophen, and muscle relaxants are all effective.

Supportive care
Return pt to light duty as soon as possible. Bed rest increases risk for atrophy of muscles and has never been shown to improve pain.
Ice, heat, massage, range-of-motion exercises, stretching, and physical therapy can all expedite recovery.
Pt should be educated on proper lifting techniques and on the red flags that would prompt further evaluation.

Pts with neurologic symptoms or epidural abscess require emergent neurosurgery/orthopedic evaluation in the ED
Consider starting high-dose corticosteroids for cauda equina or spinal cord injury.
Broad-spectrum antibiotics should be started immediately for an epidural abscess or osteomyelitis.

Disposition
Most pts can be discharged home provided they have no neurologic deficits or red flags identified on history and physical. Most will improve in 4 to 6 wks regardless of treatment provided.
Admit pts with fracture, osteomyelitis, epidural abscess, cauda equina, or having any neurologic deficits.

S — Determine the PQRST of the pain. (See Chest Pain p. 8.)
Pain along the radial aspect of the wrist suggests de Quervain's tenosynovitis.
Pain, decreased sensation, or weakness of the thumb and palm suggests carpal tunnel syndrome (CTS).

Document the pt's dominant hand
Was the pt involved in any trauma (e.g., fall, direct blow, motor vehicle crash)?
Attempt to determine position of hand and arm when the pt fell or was hit. Can predict the type of injury seen.
If a laceration or abrasion is present, document pt's last tetanus immunization.

Has the pain been gradual in onset?
CTS, de Quervain's syndrome, or chronic sprains are more likely.
Pain associated with redness and warmth should also suggest a septic joint or gout.

Is there any associated numbness or weakness?
CTS may present with both weakness and numbness, with a classic history that the pt keeps dropping things.
Fractures can impinge on or damage nerves, leading to sensory or motor weakness.

Does the pt have any other medical conditions?
Rheumatoid arthritis, pregnancy, hypothyroidism, end-stage renal disease, fibromyalgia, and diabetes are associated with an increased risk of CTS.
Osteoporosis increases the risk for bone fractures.

What medications does the pt take?
Inquire about over-the-counter medications that the pt may have tried to relieve pain.
Long-term steroid use can lead to osteoporosis and bone fractures.

Obtain a social history
Document occupation, and specifically inquire about tasks preformed at work.
Repetitive injuries or motions increase risk for CTS and de Quervain's.

O — Evaluate the pt's vital signs
Perform a physical exam
Wrist/Hand:
- Localize area of pain or tenderness. Note any bone deformity or angulation.
- Note size and shape of any lacerations or abrasions.
- Document capillary refill and pulse strength and character.
- Test passive and active range of motion of all hand joints, wrist, and elbow.
- Perform sensory exam to include radial, ulnar, and median nerve areas.
- Document strength of wrist flexors, wrist extensors, thenar and hypothenar muscle groups, interosseus, and lumbricals.

If you suspect CTS, check Phalen's and Tinel's signs.
- Phalen's is the more sensitive of the two tests.

Check Finkelstein's test:
- Have pt make a fist with his/her thumb inside and being held by the other four fingers. Ask the pt to then ulnar deviate his/her wrist. Pain along the extensor pollicis brevis and abductor pollicis longus confirms the diagnosis.

Complete a full exam. Exclude other occult trauma or disease process.

Consider obtaining x-rays of the hand and wrist
Exclude fracture. May document arthritic changes.

A Carpal Tunnel Syndrome
CTS is the most common nerve entrapment syndrome, caused by compression of the median nerve as it transverses the carpal tunnel.

De Quervain's tenosynovitis
Tenosynovitis of the abductor pollicis longus and extensor pollicis brevis tendons. Mechanism: Repetitive use of hand and wrist.

Fracture
Colles fracture: radial fracture with dorsal displacement of the distal fragment with or without ulnar styloid fracture. Mechanism: Fall on outstretched hand.
Smith fracture: opposite of Colles fracture. Radial fracture with volar displacement of the distal fragment. Mechanism: Backward fall on outstretched hand.

Differential Diagnosis
- Sprain/Contusion
- Gout
- Septic joint

P Provide effective pain relief
NSAIDs or narcotics are generally effective.
RICE therapy (Rest, Ice, Compression, Elevation)

Carpal Tunnel Syndrome
Conservative managements consists of NSAIDs, limit use of wrist, and the use of nighttime or full-time splints to keep the wrist in a neutral position.
Corticosteroid injection therapy is effective, although nerve atrophy or necrosis may occur if steroids enter the nerve sheath directly.
One-third of pts require surgery. Indications for surgery include persistent pain, motor dysfunction, or thenar eminence flattening.

De Quervain's tenosynovitis
Thumb spica, dorsal hood splint, or restricting movement of base of thumb with tape for 3 to 4 wks is effective.
Corticosteroid injection therapy is indicated for persistent pain not relieved with splints.
Refer to hand surgeon if above measures fail.

Fractures
Colles fracture has increased risk of causing acute CTS that requires immediate surgical repair.
Most fractures can be splinted with a sugar tong splint and referred to Orthopedics or a hand surgeon within 1 to 3 days. Any open fractures or fractures associated with neurologic deficits require immediate referral.

Disposition
Most pts are discharged home with follow-up arranged with their primary care provider or Orthopedics.

XI
Psychiatry

S Was the ingestion witnessed? How did it come to the attention of friends/family?
Anticipated clinical presentation, treatment options (e.g., charcoal), and lab results will depend on time of ingestion.

If pt called a friend or family member or 911, was it initially reported as a suicide attempt or accidental ingestion? Pt may change the story out of embarrassment.

What did the pt overdose on?
Attempt to quantify the actual amount ingested. May need to do a pill count and confirm with the local pharmacy the date of the last refill.

Specifically, inquire about multiple medications, illicit drugs, acetaminophen, aspirin, and alcohol.

Does the pt have a history of suicide attempts?
How has the pt attempted suicide in the past? When was the last attempt?

What other medical problems does the pt have?
Renal or liver disorders may affect the elimination and metabolism of medication/drug ingested.

What medications does the pt take on a regular basis?
Necessary to identify any drug–drug interactions.

Inquire specifically about herbal supplements and over-the-counter medications.

Obtain a social history
Important to document any history of alcohol or drug use.

Any life stressors (e.g., loss of job, fight with spouse, legal troubles) that may have triggered depression or suicidal ideation.

O Evaluate the pt's vital signs
Perform a physical exam
Constellation of symptoms will help identify a specific toxidrome.

General: Is the pt cooperative or combative? Lethargic, somnolent, or awake?

HEENT: Document size of pupils and their reactivity. Nystagmus? Dry mucous membranes? Flushing?

Lungs: Typically normal.

Cardiac: Note any tachycardia or bradycardia.

Abdomen: Note presence of bowel sounds and whether they are hypo- or hyperactive.

Extremities: Note capillary refill, color of nail beds (e.g., cherry red, cyanosis).

Neurologic: Document pt's mental status, any focal deficits.

Obtain the following labs
Electrolytes, BUN, creatinine, LFT, CBC, coags, and serum osmolarity: Typically normal. Obtain as a baseline and to exclude any other disease processes.
- Note any acidosis, anion gap, or osmolar gap.

Urine drug screen, acetaminophen, ethanol, and aspirin levels:
- Identify or confirm ingestion and degree of ingestion.

Consider obtaining drug level of any drug involved in ingestion.
- Commonly available levels include digoxin, phenobarbital, phenytoin, and valproic acid.

Obtain an ECG. Exclude any heart blocks or QT prolongation
Radiographs are typically not needed
Plain films may demonstrate a collection of pills in the stomach (e.g., bezoar).

Overdose

A History and physical exam are most important in attempting to define the ingestion. Micromedex is an excellent source to obtain information on any medication/drug, including treatment options and pill/capsule identification.

Oral hypoglycemics, β-blockers, calcium channel blockers, tricyclic antidepressants, iron, or oil of wintergreen can all be fatal to toddlers with only one or two tablets being consumed.

Consider your MUDPILES (Methanol, Urea, Diabetes ketoacidosis, Paraldehyde, Isopropyl alcohol, Lactic acidosis, Ethylene glycol, Salicylates) diagnosis with any anion gap acidosis seen. An osmolar gap may help confirm ethylene glycol, methanol, or isopropyl alcohol ingestion.

Suicide Attempt
Most pts will require psychiatric evaluation to ensure that the ingestion was not a suicide attempt.

Differential Diagnosis
- Hypoglycemia
- Hypoxia
- Cerebrovascular accident
- Sepsis
- Delirium

P **Mainstay of treatment is diligent supportive care**
Support respiration and intubate if pt is unable to protect the airway.
Provide IV hydration and ensure that the pt is not dehydrated.
If extremely combative and at risk for hurting self or others, pt will require sedation. Consider haloperidol with or without lorazepam. Some pts may require intubation and complete sedation with paralytics in order to gain control.

Consult your local poison control center or toxicologist
Consider a psychiatry consult
Consider giving activated charcoal
If pt is at risk for aspiration and will not cooperate with its administration, it is often best not to administer it.
Ideally, it should be administered within the first 2 hrs.
Late administration may help prevent enterohepatic circulation or delayed absorption, as is seen with a bezoar.

Prolonged QT duration can be treated with calcium gluconate and alkalinization
If acetaminophen overdose is suspected, the pt should ideally have N-acetylcysteine administered within 8 hrs of ingestion
Initial dose is 140 mg/kg orally, then 70 mg/kg every 4 hrs for 17 doses. IV N-acetylcysteine is not approved in the United States but is the preferred route of administration in Europe.

Disposition
All pts should be admitted for observation.

S — What prompted the pt to present to the ED?
Most common presentation is for suicidal ideation or depression.
Family/friends may bring an individual in for acting bizarrely, neglecting social obligations (e.g., job, financial obligations, family commitments), or because pt is reportedly suicidal.
Did the pt leave a note or discuss any plans on ending his/her life with anyone?

Does the pt have a history of any psychiatric illness?
Who is the psychiatrist/psychologist?
Have any of pt's medications been changed or stopped recently?

Have there been any life stressors that may be affecting the pt's mood/affect?
Recent loss of a loved one or job, marital, legal or financial difficulties

Does the pt have any other medical problems?
Depression commonly co-exists with other illnesses.
Delirium is associated with postoperative states, malnutrition, hypoglycemia, hypoxia, hepatic or renal failure, and infections.
- An exacerbation of most disease processes can cause delirium.

What medications is the pt taking?
Delirium is associated with the use of three or more medications.
A careful medication review is warranted to exclude a drug interaction as the cause of the pt's current symptoms.

Obtain a social history
Alcohol and drug history must be obtained. Acute intoxication or drug/alcohol withdrawal can prompt an ED visit for a psychiatric evaluation.

Obtain a review of symptoms
Symptom history may suggest an alternative diagnosis that is treatable and reversible.
Common symptoms associated with depression include weight loss or gain, change in appetite, depressed mood, anhedonia, sleep disturbances, feelings of worthlessness or guilt, lack of energy or psychomotor agitation, and inability to concentrate.

O — Evaluate the pt's vital signs
Ensure that the pt is hemodynamically stable and oxygenating well.

Perform a physical exam
HEENT: Note size and reactivity of pupils. Nystagmus? Mucous membranes dry or moist?
Lungs, Cardiac: Typically normal. Note any significant bradycardia or tachycardia.
Abdomen: Typically normal. Note hypo- or hyperactive bowel sounds.
Extremities: Note any evidence of self-harm (e.g., self-inflicted burns, lacerations, prior suicide attempts).
Neurologic: Assess mental status and exclude focal neurologic deficits.
Psychiatric: Evaluate mood, affect, judgment, and insight. Note any evidence of hallucinations, delusions, or suicidal or homicidal ideations. Evaluate the pt's ability to concentrate (e.g., WORLD, serial sevens). Evaluate short- and long-term memory.

Obtain the following labs
CBC, electrolytes, BUN, creatinine, urine drug screen, ethanol level:
- Exclude renal or electrolyte disturbances.
- Most psychiatric liaisons require drug and alcohol screening before their evaluation.

Consider sending a TSH if hypothyroidism is suspected.
Consider drug levels on any medication the pt takes that requires following levels.

Radiographs and ECG are generally not required
Consider obtaining a head CT if there is any question of trauma or concern for a cerebrovascular accident (CVA).

A

Mood Disorder
Includes depression, bipolar disorder, dysthymia, and cyclothymia.
Occurs in approximately 15% of the population.

Acute Psychosis
Dysfunctional thought process or behavior that can present with hallucinations, delusions, or disorganized speech and/or behavior.
Need to exclude reversible medical causes before attributing it to psychiatric cause (e.g., schizophrenia, schizoaffective disorder, brief psychotic disorder).
Common medical causes include:
- Hypoxia
- CVA
- Drug effect
- Withdrawal syndrome
- Hypoglycemia
- Liver failure
- Trauma
- Infection
- Renal failure
- Endocrine disorder

The main role of the ED physician is to exclude any medical (e.g., organic) disorder before transferring the pt to a psychiatric service.

P

Treat any underlying disorder identified
Provide supportive care
Consider providing anxiolytics if pt is very anxious.

Suture any lacerations that are identified
Update tetanus immunization if indicated.

Ensure that pt is under suicide watch if there has been a suicide attempt
Consider an involuntary psychiatric admission if pt refuses admission and you think he or she is at risk to hurt self or others.

Obtain a psychiatric consult once pt is medically cleared
Disposition
Most pts will be admitted. All pts who are suicidal or homicidal need to be detained until full evaluation is completed.
Consider discharging pts if they have close psychiatric follow-up, a close support system, have contracted for safety, and there has been no recent suicide or homicide attempt.

XII
Dermatology

Contact Dermatitis

S
When did the pt first notice the rash?
Where is the rash located?
Contact dermatitis occurs in areas that come into direct contact with the offending agent.
Eczema can occur anywhere, but atopic eczema typically involves the flexor surfaces, face, neck, and scalp.
Dishidrotic eczema tends to appear as small vesicles on the hands and feet.

Is the rash associated with any new soap, detergent, perfume, lotion, makeup, or other topical preparation?
A careful history may elicit the causative agent. The above agents can have a direct toxic effect on the skin.

Is the rash associated with any new medications or food?
Medication and food may have a direct toxic effect on the skin but is more likely to elicit an allergic reaction.

Is there a personal or family history of eczema?
Increased risk for allergic reactions and contact dermatitis

Has there been any exposure to plants or recent yard work?
Increased risk for poison ivy, poison oak, and poison sumac. The oils of the plants can persist on the skin for days, increasing the risk for secondary spread if the pt scratches.

Is the rash pruritic?
Eczema and contact dermatitis are associated with pruritus that can become very intense.

Is there any drainage, warmth, or erythema from the affected area?
Can signify a secondary infection.

Document the pt's past medical history, medication list, allergies, and social history
History of asthma or seasonal allergies increases risk of atopic eczema.

O
Evaluate the pt's vital signs
A fever should suggest a secondary infection or alternative diagnosis.

Perform a physical exam
Skin: Describe the rash. Document the size and location. Note any surrounding warmth, tenderness, or drainage that may signify a secondary infection.
- *Contact dermatitis*: Well-demarcated papules or plaques with or without overlying vesicles in the area of exposure. Vesicles may weep and crust over.
  - Classic presentation is associated with poison ivy, which tends to have linear streaks of papules with vesicles.
- *Eczema*: May have erythema, lichenification, xerosis, fissuring, and/or vesicle formation.
- *Seborrheic dermatitis*: Localized erythema with scaling skin that may appear greasy. Involves the hairy areas of the body.

Complete the physical exam.

Consider obtaining the following labs
If tinea is suspected, obtain a KOH wet prep and look for hyphae or pseudo-hyphae.
Skin biopsy can confirm diagnosis.

Skin patch testing may help elicit the causative agent. Not generally performed in the ED.
HIV: If new-onset seborrheic dermatitis is diagnosed.

Radiographs are not needed

A

Dermatitis
Contact dermatitis: Caused by an allergic or direct toxic effect of the causative agent, where it makes direct contact with the skin.
Seborrheic dermatitis: Cause is not clearly understood. Severe new onset of seborrheic dermatitis requires an evaluation for HIV.
Dishidrotic dermatitis: An intensely pruritic chronic recurrent dermatitis. Etiology is unknown. Typically involves the palms, soles, and lateral aspects of the fingers.
Atopic dermatitis: Chronic inflammatory skin disease whose etiology is not fully understood. There is a strong genetic predisposition, with 50% of affected pts reporting a family history. Most pts will have developed symptoms by the time they are 5 to 7 years old and complain of intensely pruritic erythematous patches with papules and some scaling.

Differential Diagnosis
- Cellulitis   - Psoriasis   - Impetigo
- Erysipelas   - Herpes zoster   - Tinea

P

Avoid causative agent if identified
Mainstay of therapy if possible. Ivy Block is an over-the-counter preparation that is applied like suntan lotion and can help reduce the risk of poison ivy when outdoor activities make exposure likely.

Provide symptomatic relief of pruritus
- Oatmeal baths   - Antihistamines   - Moisturizing creams or ointments

Consider topical steroids
Can be effective for nonspecific dermatitis and dishidrotic dermatitis.
Topical steroids should be used for 2 to 3 wks. Prolonged use can cause skin atrophy and hypopigmentation.

Consider oral steroids
Indicated for contact dermatitis and severe cases of dishidrotic dermatitis and atopic dermatitis.
Poison ivy typically requires a long 2- to 3-week course. The short course offered by a methylprednisolone dose pack typically results in a recurrence or treatment failure.

Seborrheic dermatitis responds well to antiseborrheic shampoos with ketoconazole, pyrithione, selenium, or zinc

Disposition
All pts can be discharged home, unless they require IV antibiotics for a secondary infection.
All pts should follow up with their primary care provider, who can refer to Dermatology if pts do not respond to the above treatment.

Urticaria

S **When did the rash occur?**
An episode of urticaria, hives, typically lasts less then 6 hrs and should completely resolve by 36 hrs. Vasculitis should be considered if lesions last more than 24 hrs.

Does the rash itch or is it painful?
Urticaria is pruritic; if the lesions are painful, vasculitis should be considered.

Is the outbreak associated with a particular activity, food item consumed, medication taken, or insect bite?
Urticaria is often associated with an allergic reaction, but it may also be triggered by stress (emotional or physical), cold temperatures, or insect bites.

Does the pt have any difficulty breathing or swallowing?
Ensure that there is no airway swelling that can compromise respirations.

Does the pt have any other medical problems?
Cancer, lupus, Sjögren's syndrome, thyroid disorders, and cryoglobulinemia may present with urticaria as their presenting symptom.

What medications is the pt taking?
Determine if hives are temporally related to taking any medication.
Determine whether any medications are new or have been recently refilled. If medication was newly filled, pt may have received the wrong medication or a new formulation and be having a reaction to one of the inactive components of the tablet/capsule.
Antibiotics, aspirin, hormones, and NSAIDs are the most common drugs implicated.
IV vancomycin that is administered too fast can result in Redman syndrome and hives.

Obtain an allergy list and social history
Sulfa allergies are fairly common, and many medications (e.g., all diuretics except ethacrynic acid, celecoxib) contain sulfa that may be missed when initially prescribed.

Is there a family history of urticaria?
Familial cold autoinflammatory syndrome and Muckle-Wells syndrome are two rare genetic causes of urticaria that have mutations in cryopyrin, a protein involved in the early stages of inflammation.

Obtain a review of symptoms
Fever, weight loss, arthritic pain, or hot or cold intolerance may suggest a secondary cause of urticaria (e.g., lupus, cancer, or thyroid abnormality).

O **Perform a physical exam**
Skin:
- Note distribution of urticaria (e.g., raised, demarcated, erythematous papules with central pallor that may coalesce into plaques).
- Note any dermatographism (urticaria that results from lightly scratching or writing on the skin with a blunt object).

Lungs: Document any wheezing or respiratory distress.
Complete a full physical exam.

Consider obtaining the following labs
TSH: If history suggests thyroid disorder.
ESR: May be elevated in lupus or cancer.
CBC: Typically normal, although WBC differential may show eosinophilia.

A Urticaria

May affect up to 25% of the population.
Secondary causes include lupus, cryoglobulinemia, and thyroid disease.
Mediated by the cutaneous mast cell in the superficial dermis.
Angioedema may coexist in up to 50% of pts with urticaria.
Chronic urticaria may develop in approximately 30% of cases. Diagnosed as chronic urticaria if recurrences go on for more than 6 wks; 40% of pts with urticaria beyond 6 months will still have symptoms at 10 years.

Urticarial Vasculitis
Associated with autoimmune disorders (e.g., lupus, Sjögren's).
Typical lesion is painful, lasts > 24 hrs, leaves a residual pigmentation, and resists corticosteroid therapy.

Differential Diagnosis
- Contact dermatitis
- Cellulitis
- Insect bite
- Eczema
- Folliculitis

P Provide symptomatic relief
Pruritus can be treated with oatmeal baths, antihistamines, and moisturizing cream.

Pharmacologic therapy
Antihistamines are the mainstay of therapy.
- H_1 receptor blockers (e.g., diphenhydramine, loratadine, hydroxyzine) in combination with an H_2 receptor blocker (e.g., ranitidine, famotidine, cimetidine) are effective in improving rash and resolving the lesions.

Doxepin, an antidepressant and antihistamine with H_1 and H_2 receptor action, has also been very effective in eliminating symptoms. This drug is up to seven times more potent than hydroxyzine in suppressing wheal and flare responses.
Corticosteroids are extremely effective in resistant cases or for treatment of chronic urticaria.
Epinephrine should be reserved for severe cases that are associated with angioedema and respiratory distress.

Disposition
Most pts can be discharged home and follow up with their primary care provider.
Admit pts who have angioedema that is associated with respiratory distress or who have a risk of developing respiratory distress.

XIII

Pediatrics

S **Determine the PQRST of the pain.** (See Chest Pain p. 8.)
Depending on the age of the pt, this may be impossible.

When did the parents notice the child having pain? How did they know the child was uncomfortable?
Establish the time course and extent of pain.
Child may appear well in the ED, but intermittent severe pain with normal exam and activity between episodes is seen with intussusception.

Is the pain associated with nausea and vomiting?
May be secondary to gastroenteritis, but can also be caused by a complete obstruction.
Is the emesis associated with meals and projectile? Pyloric stenosis typically presents between 2 weeks and 2 months of life in first-born males, with projectile emesis occurring after meals.

Has the pt had a fever?
Associated with appendicitis and viral syndromes.

When was the pt's last bowel movement?
Abdominal pain caused by constipation is common.
Inquire about diarrhea, jelly-like stools, or bloody stools. Can be seen in partial bowel obstructions, volvulus, or intussusception.

Has the pt had any prior abdominal surgeries?
Increases risk of obstruction from adhesions.

Has the pt been involved in any trauma or abuse?
Increased risk of solid organ injury with blunt trauma.
Falling off bicycle and hitting handlebars is classically associated with intestinal rupture or pancreatic contusion.

If a female adolescent, is the pt of reproductive age and/or sexually active?
Ectopic pregnancy and pelvic inflammatory disease (PID) need to be considered in the differential.

Obtain the pt's past medical history, medication list, allergies, and social history
Obtain a review of symptoms
May suggest an alternative diagnosis.
Polyuria, polydipsia, and weight loss may suggest diabetes and diabetic ketoacidosis as the cause of abdominal pain.

O **Evaluate the pt's vital signs**
Note temperature. Tachycardia is the first sign of shock.

Perform a physical exam
Abdomen: Note any tenderness, rebound tenderness, or peritoneal signs.
- Palpate for masses. Olive-shaped mass in the epigastrum is classic for pyloric stenosis but rarely felt.
- Palpate for umbilical and inguinal hernias with incarceration.

GU: Palpate testicles and ensure that they are descended. Consider testicular torsion as cause of pain.
Rectal: Guaiac stool.

Gyn: Examine adolescents to exclude PID, ovarian cyst.
Complete a full physical exam.

Obtain the following labs
CBC: Exclude anemia and elevated WBC.
Electrolytes, Glucose: Exclude electrolyte disturbance, acidosis, and diabetes.
Urinalysis, BUN, Creatinine: Exclude infection and renal disease.
LFT, amylase, lipase: Exclude liver and pancreatic disease.
β-hCG: Exclude pregnancy.

Consider obtaining the following x-rays
CXR: Exclude pneumonia and bowel perforation, as evidenced by air under diaphragm.
Acute Abdominal Series: Exclude obstruction as shown by air-fluid levels, dilated bowel loops.
Abdominal CT Scan: Test of choice. Can demonstrate appendicitis, volvulus, renal nephrolithiasis, and pyloric stenosis. May demonstrate intussusception.
Air-contrast enema: Test of choice for volvulus and intussusception. Can be diagnostic and therapeutic for intussusception.
Ultrasound: Can diagnose appendicitis, intussusception, pregnancy, ectopic pregnancy, testicular torsion, and pyloric stenosis.

A ### Abdominal Pain
Children may somatize their emotional distress as abdominal pain.
It is extremely important to listen to the parent's account of the child's symptoms because many disorders (e.g., intussusception, volvulus) have intermittent pain, and child may appear well in the ED.

Differential Diagnosis
- Appendicitis	- Intussusception	- Volvulus
- Renal colic	- Gastroenteritis	- Constipation
- Somatization disorder	- Pancreatitis	- Child abuse
- UTI	- PID	- Ectopic pregnancy

P **Obtain surgical consult immediately for intussusception, volvulus, appendicitis, incarcerated hernia, ectopic pregnancy, or perforated bowel**
If diagnosis is unsure, consider second surgical opinion.

Pain relief remains controversial
Multiple studies have shown that narcotics do not hinder the ability to diagnose the cause of abdominal pain, nor do they increase the rate of complications. However, the dogma has been to withhold pain medication until the child has been evaluated by surgery.
- Pain medications may help increase the sensitivity of your physical exam, by allowing the child to cooperate with the exam and decrease voluntary guarding.

Disposition
Pts whose pain has resolved and workup has excluded any serious pathology can be discharged home after a period of observation in the ED.
All other pts should be admitted for serial abdominal exams or surgery.

Febrile Seizures

S

How long did the seizure last? Who witnessed the seizure?
Have witness describe the seizure activity, if any, that was witnessed.

Has the child been sick or had a fever?
Febrile seizures are common in children 6 months to 5 years.

Was the child involved in a trauma or suffered a head injury?
Will need to exclude an intracerebral hemorrhage or contusion as cause of seizure.

Does the child have a known seizure disorder?
Ensure that the child has been compliant with seizure medications, and ascertain how often the child has seizures, and if this seizure was different from normal seizure.

Has the child started any new medication or ingested anything?
Seizure can be caused by a medication reaction or be secondary to toxic ingestion or intoxication.

Has the child had a headache or any neurologic deficits?
Severe or chronic headaches and/or neurologic deficits with seizures requires an evaluation for brain tumors.

Obtain a complete past medical history, medication list, allergy list, and social history
Obtain a family history
Inquire about any history of metabolic disorders or seizure disorders.

Obtain a review of symptoms
Rhinorrhea, cough, ear pain, and fever suggest a febrile seizure.

O

Evaluate the pt's vital signs
Note temperature and obtain a pulse oximetry to ensure adequate oxygenation.

Perform a physical exam
HEENT: Inspect for signs of trauma. Visualize tympanic membranes to exclude trauma and infection. Inspect nares for rhinorrhea and cerebrospinal fluid leak. Palpate neck for tenderness, bone deformity or stepoff, and adenopathy.
Lungs, Cardiac: Typically normal. Auscultate for signs of pneumonia.
Abdomen: Typically normal.
Extremities: Evaluate for trauma.
Neurologic: Evaluate cranial nerves, sensation, and motor function of all limbs, and mental status. Note any deficits.

Obtain the following labs
CBC: Exclude anemia or increased WBC as sign of infection.
Electrolytes, glucose, BUN, creatinine: Exclude electrolyte disturbance, renal dysfunction.
Consider obtaining:
- Toxic screen and alcohol level if intoxication is suspected
- Drug levels of antiseizure medication the child is on
- Lumbar puncture if central nervous system infection is suspected

Consider obtaining a head CT scan if there is a history of trauma, abuse, neurologic deficit, or chronic or severe headaches
Exclude underlying brain tumor, intracerebral hemorrhage, and skull fracture.

EEGs are generally not obtained in the ED

A **Febrile Seizure**
Usually a generalized seizure that lasts < 15 minutes with no residual neurologic deficits
Often seen when temperature is increasing rapidly but can also occur as the pt's fever is declining.
A complex febrile seizure lasts > 15 minutes, or multiple generalized seizures in 1 hour, or a seizure with residual focal neurologic deficits.
Risk of developing epilepsy is only slightly higher than the general population.

Infantile Spasm (IS)
An epilepsy syndrome of infancy and early childhood with onset of first seizure typically between 3 to 6 months
The typical pattern of IS is a sudden bending forward and stiffening of the body, arms, and legs, although there can also be arching of the torso. Spasms tend to last for 1 to 5 seconds and occur in clusters, ranging from 2 to 100 spasms at a time.
25% of infants with IS will have tuberous sclerosis.

Epilepsy
Differential Diagnosis
- Drug withdrawal
- Movement disorder
- Meningitis
- Hypoglycemia

P **Provide supportive care**
Ensure that child maintains airway and does not become hypoxic.
Protect child from harm when seizing.

Febrile Seizures
No specific treatment is needed other than aggressive management of the fever.
Treat any underlying infection.
There is no role for antiepileptics.

Infantile Spasm
Refer to a pediatric neurologist.
Children are often treated with steroids, corticotropin, or antiepileptic medications.
Should be tested for tuberous sclerosis.

Epilepsy
If newly diagnosed, refer to pediatrician or pediatric neurologist.
Most specialists will not start antiepileptics with a single seizure.

Disposition
Most pts with febrile seizure and epilepsy can be discharged home provided their parents are comfortable and they have follow-up with their pediatrician.
Children who are newly diagnosed with infantile spasm will probably be admitted to facilitate evaluation and treatment. Consult the pediatrician.

Fever of Unknown Origin — Pediatrics

S

Is there a documented fever at home or in the ED?
If caregiver has documented a temperature > 38°C, a full evaluation is required in the ED regardless of what the temperature is in the ED.

Has the child demonstrated any localizing signs (e.g., ear tugging, cough, rhinorrhea, pain with urination)?
Attempt to localize the source of infection. In children < 3 months, this is extremely difficult.

Has there been any nausea, vomiting, or diarrhea?
Can occur with any systemic illness and increases the risk for dehydration.

Has there been any change in the child's activity level or amount of sleep?
Children will typically become lethargic and sleep more when they have a fever.

Has there been any change in the number of wet diapers or trips to the bathroom today?
Used as a guide to ascertain whether the child is dehydrated.

Is the child being fed formula or breast milk?
Breast milk decreases the risk of recurrent infections.

Obtain a past medical history
Ask specifically if there were any prenatal or delivery complications.
Was the pt preterm, and if so, did he or she require a NICU stay, and for how long?

Obtain a medication list and allergy list
Ask specifically about any antipyretics (e.g., acetaminophen, aspirin, ibuprofen) or antibiotics the pt may have received.

Obtain a social history
Document exposure to second-hand smoke, which increases the risk for ear and respiratory infections.
Does the child attend day care? Increased risk for frequent viral illnesses.

Obtain a family history
Document any history of genetic disorders (e.g., cystic fibrosis) or immune deficiencies.

O

Evaluate the pt's vital signs. Obtain a rectal temperature. Note SpO_2.

Perform a physical exam
General: Note activity level and attentiveness.
HEENT: Note ability to form tears. Lack of tear formation suggests dehydration.
  Inspect ears, nares, and neck. Note any otitis media or externa, signs of viral illness, or neck stiffness.
Lungs: Auscultate for wheezing and consolidation.
Cardiac: Note tachycardia or murmurs.
Abdomen: Note tenderness, distention, or rashes.
Extremities: Note any cyanosis or rash.
Skin: Note skin turgor or rash.

Obtain the following labs
CBC: WBC > 15,000 suggests a bacterial infection.
Urinalysis: Leukocyte esterase, nitrite, or WBC > 5 suggests urinary tract infection (UTI).
Blood culture: Exclude occult bacterial infection.

Obtain a lumbar puncture in all children < 30 days, high-risk children > 30 but < 90 days, and all toxic-appearing children
Low risk is defined as a previously healthy infant with no chronic medical illness who appears well, WBC on CBC > 5000 and < 15,000 with normal differential, urinalysis, and CXR. If cerebrospinal fluid (CSF) was sent, WBC < 8 WBC/mm^3 with no organisms.

Obtain a CXR. Exclude pneumonia.

A **Fever**
Guidelines for treating children with fever are age specific.
The high rate of occult bacteremia in newborns (< 30 days old) requires that all newborns receive a full workup and that empiric broad-spectrum antibiotics be started.
Most fevers are caused by a self-limited viral infection.
Common bacterial causes include *E. coli*, *H. influenzae*, Group B *Streptococcus*, *Listeria*, and *N. meningitides*.

Differential Diagnosis
- Viral syndrome   - Otitis media   - Pneumonia
- Bronchitis   - UTI   - Meningitis/Encephalitis

P **Provide supportive care**
Antipyretics for fever (e.g., acetaminophen or ibuprofen). Avoid aspirin.
IV or PO hydration if signs of dehydration are present. IV fluid challenge is 20 cc/kg.

Children < 30 days old
Admit.
Start broad-spectrum antibiotics that cover *Listeria*, *E. coli*, and Group B *Streptococcus*.
• Ampicillin plus cefotaxime or ceftriaxone plus gentamycin

Children > 30 days old and < 90 days old
Admit high-risk and toxic-appearing children. Start IV cefotaxime or ceftriaxone.
For low-risk or well-appearing children, discuss discharge planning with pediatrician. Some pediatricians will treat with a single dose of ceftriaxone and await culture results; others prefer to not treat empirically with antibiotics. If antibiotics are going to be given, a lumbar puncture should be done beforehand to exclude occult meningitis.

Children > 3 months old
Admit toxic-appearing children and start empiric antibiotics (e.g., ceftriaxone).
Well-appearing children can be discharged home. Generally withhold antibiotics if temperature is < 39°C, but discuss each child with the pediatrician to ensure coordination of care.

Disposition
Children discharged home must follow up with their pediatrician with 48 hrs.

Gastroenteritis

S **What are the child's current symptoms?**
Common symptoms include:
- Nausea/vomiting
- Diarrhea
- Fever
- Tenesmus
- Abdominal pain
- Headache

How long has the child been ill?
Was the onset of the illness associated with any travel, new foods, or formula?
- Food and formula suggest a food allergy.
- Travel increases the risk of parasitic, viral, and bacterial infections.

If the child is having abdominal pain, quantify its timing and severity
Intermittent, severe abdominal pain with nausea/vomiting can be seen with intussusception and volvulus.

Quantify the amount of vomiting and/or diarrhea
Assess the pt's risk for dehydration.

Does anything trigger the vomiting?
Vomiting after meals suggests intestinal obstruction.
Inquire about the amount and frequency of the child's feeding to exclude overfeeding from the differential.

Have there been any blood or "coffee grounds" in the emesis?
Exclude a gastrointestinal bleed.

Does the child have any other medical problems?
Document any prenatal or delivery complications.

What medications has the child been taking?
Inquire specifically about over-the-counter antidiarrhea medications.
Any new medications (e.g., antibiotics) may suggest an adverse drug reaction.

Obtain an allergy list, social history, and family history
Ascertain if any other family contacts are ill; suggests an infectious cause.

Obtain a review of symptoms

O **Evaluate the pt's vital signs**
Tachycardia and hypotension are ominous signs of severe dehydration.

Perform a physical exam
General: Is the child's attentiveness appropriate for age? Lethargic or somnolent?
HEENT: Typically normal. Lack of tears and dry mucous membranes are seen with dehydration.
Lungs, Cardiac: Typically normal. May have tachycardia.
Abdomen: Note any tenderness, rebound, or abnormal bowel sounds.
Rectal: Check guaiac to exclude blood in stool.
Skin: Evaluate skin turgor.

Consider obtaining the following labs if child is ill appearing
CBC: Exclude anemia or significantly elevated WBC. Eosinophilia suggests parasitic infection.
Electrolytes, BUN, creatinine, glucose: Exclude electrolyte disorder, renal insufficiency, and hypoglycemia, hyperglycemia.
Urinalysis: Ketones and high specific gravity support dehydration. Exclude urinary tract infection.

Consider sending stool for C. *difficile*, ova and parasites, rotavirus, and culture
Consider obtaining acute abdominal series or CT of abdomen/pelvis if concerned about possible obstruction
Exclude obstruction, volvulus, and intussusception.

A ### Gastroenteritis
Extremely common, with up to 30 million cases per year in the United States.
Most commonly caused by a virus (e.g., Rotavirus, enteroviruses, Norwalk virus, or adenoviruses).
Bloody diarrhea should suggest a bacterial cause from *Campylobacter, Clostridium difficile, E. coli O157, Salmonella, Shigella,* or *Yersinia*.
- Other bacterial causes include *Vibrio, Bacillus cereus, Listeria,* and *Staphylococcus aureus.*

Common parasitic causes include *Cryptosporidium, E. histolytica,* and *Giardia.*
Most cases are self-limited and require only supportive care.

Differential Diagnosis
- Volvulus - Intussusception - Lactose intolerance
- Overfeeding - Pyloric stenosis - Malabsorption syndrome

P ### Provide supportive care
If child is dehydrated, attempt oral rehydration with commercially available oral electrolyte solutions.
IV hydration with normal saline or lactated Ringer's 20 cc/kg in those pts who do not tolerate oral therapy.
Correct any electrolyte abnormalities noted on labs.
Avoid use of antidiarrhea medications that contain opiates or anticholinergics.

Treat the underlying infection if identified
Most bacterial infections do not require antibiotics, and antibiotics may prolong the carrier state and increase the risk of hemolytic-uremic syndrome in *E. coli* infections.
- Administer antibiotics in toxic-appearing children, children with a history of immunocompromise, or those younger than 6 months.

Most parasitic infections can be treated with metronidazole.

Disposition
Well-appearing children who have demonstrated their ability to tolerate oral hydration can be discharged home with close follow-up with their pediatrician.
Admit ill, toxic-appearing children, and those who are unable to tolerate oral hydration.

Index

A
Abdominal aortic aneurysm, 58–59
Abdominal pain, 60, 68, 78
   in children, 188–189
Abortion, spontaneous, 134–135
Abscess
   peritonsillar, 99
   retropharyngeal, 99
   tubo-ovarian, 127
ACE inhibitor, in congestive heart failure, 11
Acetaminophen overdoses, 177
N-Acetylcysteine, 177
Achilles tendon rupture, 161
Acid burns, 162–163
Acidosis, anion gap, 177
Acute renal failure, 104–105
Adenosine challenge, in palpitations, 19
Alcohol abuse
   anemia and, 28
   gastrointestinal bleeding and, 74
   hepatitis and, 76
   hypoglycemia and, 38, 39
Alkali burns, 162–163
Allergy, 184–185
Altered mental status, 142–143
Alveolar osteitis, 101
Amanita poisoning, 76
Ammonia, 77
Amyotrophic lateral sclerosis, 155
Anemia, 28–29
Aneurysm, aortic, 58–59
Angina, 8–9
   unstable, 22–23
Angiography
   in ischemic bowel, 78
   in pulmonary embolism, 55
Animal bites, 158–159
Anion gap acidosis, 177
Ankle
   fracture of, 161
   sprain of, 160–161
Antacids, in gastroesophageal reflux disease, 73
Anterior draw test, 160
Antibiotics
   in appendicitis, 61
   in bowel obstruction, 63
   in corneal abrasion, 89
   in diarrhea, 67
   in gastroenteritis, 195
   in meningitis, 147
   in pelvic inflammatory disease, 131
   in pneumonia, 49
   in urinary tract infection, 115
   in vulvovaginitis, 139
Anticoagulation, in pulmonary embolism, 55
Antihistamines, in urticaria, 185
Aorta
   aneurysm of, 58–59
   dissection of, 2–3
Appendicitis, 60–61
Arrhythmias, 6–7, 19
   in aortic dissection, 3
   reperfusion, 17
Aspirin, in myocardial infarction, 17
Asthma, 42–43
Atopic dermatitis, 183
Atrial fibrillation, 19
Atrial flutter, 19
Atropine, in bradycardia, 5
Avulsion, tooth, 100–101

B
Bacterial infection. *See* Infection
Bacterial vaginosis, 138, 139
Beta-blocker
   in myocardial infarction, 17
   overdose of, 5
Bicarbonate, in diabetic ketoacidosis, 37
Biliary colic, 65
Biliary disease, 64–65
Bismuth subsalicylate, 67
Bites, 116, 158–159
Bleeding
   diverticular, 69
   gastrointestinal, 74–75
   nasal, 92–93
   vaginal, 136–137
Blood pressure, in aortic dissection, 3
Blood transfusion
   in anemia, 29
   in gastrointestinal bleeding, 75
   in sickle cell crisis, 33
Bowel
   ischemic, 78–79
   obstruction of, 62–63
Bradycardia, 4–5
Brandt-Daroff maneuver, 153
Bronchodilator, in chronic obstructive pulmonary disease, 45
Brudzinski sign, 146
B-type natriuretic peptide, in congestive heart failure, 11, 44
Burns, 162–163

C

Calcium channel blocker, overdose of, 5
Calculi, renal, 112–113
Candida infection, 138, 139
Cardiac arrest, 6–7
Cardioversion, in palpitations, 19
Carpal tunnel syndrome, 173
Cerebrovascular accident, aortic dissection and, 2
Cervicitis, gonococcal, 119
Chancroid, 119
Chemical burns, 162–163
Chest pain, 8–9, 22–23
Chest tube, 47
Chest x-ray
　in acute renal failure, 105
　in aortic dissection, 2
　in asthma, 43
　in cardiac arrest, 7
　in chest pain, 9, 22
　in chronic obstructive pulmonary disease, 44
　in congestive heart failure, 10
　in dysphagia, 90
　in endocarditis, 12
　in esophageal foreign body, 70
　in gastroesophageal reflux disease, 72
　in hypertensive crisis, 14
　in palpitations, 18
　in pleural effusion, 46
　in pneumonia, 48
　in pneumothorax, 50–51
　in pulmonary edema, 52
　in pulmonary embolism, 54
　in sickle cell disease, 33
Children
　abdominal pain in, 188–189
　febrile seizures in, 190–191
　fever of unknown origin in, 192–193
　gastroenteritis in, 194–195
Chlamydia infection, 119
Cholangitis, 65
Cholecystectomy, 65
Cholecystitis, 64–65
Choledocholithiasis, 65
Cholelithiasis, 65
Chronic obstructive pulmonary disease, 44–45
Cigarette smoking, cessation of, 45
Clindamycin, in vulvovaginitis, 139
Clopidogrel, in myocardial infarction, 17
Clotrimazole, in *Candida* infection, 139
Cluster headache, 145
Coin ingestion, 70–71
Colic, biliary, 65
Colles fracture, 173
Colonoscopy, in ischemic bowel, 79

Computed tomography
　in abdominal aortic aneurysm, 58
　in aortic dissection, 3
　in appendicitis, 61
　in biliary disease, 64
　in bowel obstruction, 63
　in diverticulitis, 68
　in febrile seizures, 190
　in foreign-body ingestion, 71
　in head injury, 167
　in headache, 145
　in hypertensive crisis, 14
　in ischemic bowel, 78
　in low back pain, 171
　in pleural effusion, 46
　in pneumothorax, 51
　in seizures, 149
　in sickle cell disease, 33
　in stroke, 150
　in syncope, 21
　in vertigo, 153
Concussion, 167
Congestive heart failure, 10–11
Conjunctivitis, 86–87
Consciousness, loss of, 166
Contact dermatitis, 182–183
Contact lenses, 86, 88
Corneal abrasion, 88–89
Corticosteroids
　in asthma, 43
　in chronic obstructive pulmonary disease, 45
　in dermatitis, 183
　in meningitis, 147
　in urticaria, 185
Costochondritis, 9
C-peptide, 38
Creatine kinase, in myocardial infarction, 16–17
Cremasteric reflex, 120
Cullen's sign, 80
Cyst, ovarian, 126–127

D

Dancer's fracture, 161
Deep venous thrombosis, 24–25
Defibrillation, 6
Dehydration, 21
Delirium, 142–143
Dementia, 142–143
Depression, 178–179
DeQuervain's tenosynovitis, 173
Dermatitis
　atopic, 183
　contact, 182–183

dyshidrotic, 183
seborrheic, 182, 183
Dextrose, in hypoglycemia, 39
Diabetic ketoacidosis, 36–37
Dialysis, 105
Diarrhea, 66–67
Digoxin, overdose of, 5
Diverticulitis, 68–69
Diverticulosis, 74
Dix-Hallpike maneuver, 152
Dizziness, 152–153
Dobutamine, in congestive heart failure, 11
Dopamine, in congestive heart failure, 11
Doxipen, in urticaria, 185
Dressing, wound, 169
Drug overdose, 176–177
Duke criteria, 13
Dyshidrotic dermatitis, 183
Dysphagia, 72, 90–91

E

Ear
 examination of, 94, 96
 foreign body in, 94
 infection of, 94–97
Eaton-Lambert syndrome, 155
Echocardiography
 in congestive heart failure, 11
 in endocarditis, 12
 in pulmonary embolism, 55
 in syncope, 21
Ectopic pregnancy, 124–125
Eczema, 182
Edema, pulmonary, 52–53
Effusion, pleural, 46–47
Electrocardiography
 in acute renal failure, 105
 in aortic dissection, 2
 in bradycardia, 4–5
 in cardiac arrest, 7
 in chest pain, 8, 22
 in chronic obstructive pulmonary disease, 45
 in congestive heart failure, 10
 in endocarditis, 12
 in gastroesophageal reflux disease, 72
 in gastrointestinal bleeding, 75
 in heart block, 4–5
 in hypertensive crisis, 14
 in myocardial infarction, 16
 in palpitations, 18
 in pulmonary edema, 52
 in rhabdomyolysis, 117
Electrolytes
 in diabetic ketoacidosis, 37
 in palpitations, 18

Ellis classification, 100–101
Embolism, pulmonary, 25, 54–55
Endocarditis, 12–13
Endoscopy, in foreign-body ingestion, 71
Enzymes, cardiac, 16–17, 23
Epididymitis, 106–107
Epidural hemorrhage, 167
Epiglottitis, 98, 99
Epilepsy, 191
Epinephrine
 in bradycardia, 5
 in urticaria, 185
Epistaxis, 92–93
Epley maneuver, 153
Esmolol, in hypertensive crisis, 15
Esophagus, foreign body in, 70–71, 90–91
Estrogen, in vaginal bleeding, 137
Eyes
 examination of, 86, 88
 irrigation of, 89

F

Fallopian tube, abscess of, 127
Febrile seizures, 190–191
Femoral hernia, 108
Fever of unknown origin, 192–193
Finkelstein's test, 172
Fluconazole, in *Candida* infection, 139
Fluid therapy
 in anemia, 29
 in biliary colic, 65
 in bowel obstruction, 63
 in diabetic ketoacidosis, 37
 in diarrhea, 67
 in gastrointestinal bleeding, 75
 in rhabdomyolysis, 117
Food
 esophageal blockage with, 71, 91
 in gastroesophageal reflux disease, 72
Food poisoning, in children, 194–195
Foreign body
 conjunctival, 89
 ear, 94
 ingestion of, 70–71
Fracture, 164–165
 ankle, 161
 foot, 161
 tooth, 100–101
 wrist, 173

G

Gastric lavage, 74
Gastritis, 74
Gastroenteritis, in children, 194–195
Gastroesophageal reflux disease, 8, 72–73

Gastrointestinal bleeding, 74–75
Genital herpes, 119
Genital warts, 119
Glossitis, 28
Glucagon, in hypoglycemia, 39
Glucose, blood, 38
Gonococcal infection, 119
Grey-Turner's sign, 80

H

H_2 blocker, in gastrointestinal bleeding, 75
Hampton's hump, 54
Head injury, 166–167
Headache, 144–145
Heart block, 4–5
Heart failure, 10–11
Helicobacter pylori infection, 82, 83
Heliox, in asthma, 43
Hematoma, in head injury, 167
Hemophilus influenza vaccine, 98
Hemorrhage
    cerebral, 150–151
    splinter, 12
Hemostasis, for nose bleed, 93
Heparin, in myocardial infarction, 17
Hepatitis, 76–77
Hepatobiliary nuclear scan, in biliary disease, 64
Hernia, 108–109
Herpes infection, genital, 119
Hydrocele, 110–111
Hydroxyurea, in sickle cell crisis, 33
Hyperemesis gravidarum, 128
Hypertensive crisis, 14–15
Hypertensive urgency, 15
Hypoglycemia, 21, 38–39

I

Idiopathic thrombocytopenic purpura, 30–31
Incisional hernia, 109
Infantile spasm, 191
Infection
    appendiceal, 60–61
    bite-related, 159
    conjunctival, 86–87
    ear, 94–97
    fallopian tube, 127
    gastrointestinal, in children, 194–195
    meningeal, 146–147
    ovarian, 127
    sexual assault and, 132–133
    sexually transmitted, 118–119
    urinary tract, 114–115
    vulvovaginal, 138–139
Inguinal hernia, 108

Insulin
    blood, 38
    in diabetic ketoacidosis, 37
Iron-deficiency anemia, 29
Irrigation
    eye, 89
    wound, 169
Ischemia
    cerebral, 150–151
    intestinal, 78–79
    myocardial, 6, 7, 16–17

J

Janeway lesions, 12
Jones fracture, 161

K

Kernig's sign, 147
Ketoacidosis, diabetic, 36–37
Kidney stones, 112–113

L

Laceration, 168–169
Laryngoscopy, in foreign-body ingestion, 71
Loperamide, 67
Low back pain, 170–171
Lumbar puncture
    in fever of unknown origin, 193
    in headache, 145
    in meningitis, 147
    in stroke, 150

M

Magnesium sulfate, in asthma, 43
Magnetic resonance imaging
    in aortic dissection, 3
    in low back pain, 171
    in venous thrombosis, 25
    in vertigo, 153
Mallory-Weiss tear, 74
Meningitis, 146–147
Menorrhagia, 137
Mental status, altered, 142–143
Meperidine, in sickle cell crisis, 33
Metered-dose inhaler, in asthma, 43
Metronidazole, in vulvovaginitis, 139
Metrorrhagia, 137
Miconazole, in *Candida* infection, 139
Migraine headache, 145
Miscarriage, 134–135
Mood disorder, 178–179
Morphine
    in myocardial infarction, 17
    in sickle cell crisis, 33
Multiple sclerosis, 155

Index

Murphy's sign, 64
Myasthenia gravis, 155
Myocardial infarction, 6, 7, 16–17

N
Nausea
   in bowel obstruction, 63
   headache and, 145
Nebulizer, in asthma, 43
Nephrolithiasis, 112–113
Neurologic examination, 166
Nitroglycerin, in myocardial infarction, 17
Nitroprusside, in hypertensive crisis, 15
Nonketotic hyperosmolar coma, 37
Nosebleeds, 92–93

O
Octreotide, in gastrointestinal bleeding, 75
Odynophagia, 72
Orchitis, 107
Osler's nodes, 12
Osteitis, alveolar, 101
Otitis externa, 94–95
Otitis media, 96–97
Ovary
   abscess of, 127
   cyst of, 126–127
   torsion of, 126–127
Oxygen saturation, in chest pain, 9
Oxygen therapy
   in asthma, 43
   in chronic obstructive pulmonary disease, 45
   in congestive heart failure, 11
   in pneumonia, 48
   in sickle cell crisis, 33

P
Pain
   abdominal, 188–189
   chest, 8–9
   epididymal, 106
   low back, 170–171
   wrist, 172–173
Palpitations, 18–19
Pancreatitis, 80–81
Peak flow, in asthma, 43
Pelvic inflammatory disease, 130–131
Peptic ulcer disease, 74, 82–83
Percutaneous coronary angioplasty, 17
Peritonsillar abscess, 99
Petechiae, 12
Phalen's sign, 172
Pharyngitis, 98–99
Pharynx, examination of, 98
Phenazopyridine, 115

Pleural effusion, 46–47
Pleurisy, 9
Pneumocystis carinii pneumonia, 48
Pneumonia, 48–49
Pneumothorax, 50–51
Poison ivy, 183
Pregnancy, 128–129
   ectopic, 124–125
   loss of, 134–135
   sexual assault and, 133
Premature ventricular contractions, 19
Progesterone, in vaginal bleeding, 137
Proton pump inhibitor, in gastrointestinal bleeding, 75
Psychiatric evaluation, 178–179
Psychosis, evaluation for, 178–179
Pulmonary edema, 52–53
Pulmonary embolism, 25, 54–55
Pulseless electrical activity, 6–7
Pyelonephritis, 114–115

R
Rabies vaccine, 159
Ranson's criteria, 81
Rash, 182–183
   urticarial, 184–185
Renal failure, 104–105
Retropharyngeal abscess, 99
Rhabdomyolysis, 116–117
Roth spots, 12

S
Seborrheic dermatitis, 182, 183
Seizures, 148–149
   febrile, 190–191
Semont maneuver, 153
Sexual assault, 132–133
Sexually transmitted diseases, 118–119
Sickle cell disease, 32–33
Sigmoidoscopy, in ischemic bowel, 79
Sinus bradycardia, 4–5
Smith fracture, 173
Spasm, infantile, 191
Spontaneous abortion, 134–135
Sprain, ankle, 160–161
Stones, renal, 112–113
Straight leg raise, 170
Stroke, 150–151
Subdural hemorrhage, 167
Substance abuse, overdose with, 176–177
Suicide attempt, 176–177
   evaluation for, 178–179
Supraventricular tachycardia, 19
Swallowing, difficulty in, 90–91

Syncope, 20–21
Syphilis, 119

T

Tachycardia
 in aortic dissection, 3
 supraventricular, 19
 ventricular, 6–7, 19
Talar tilt test, 160
Tension headache, 145
Tension pneumothorax, 50, 51
Terconazole, in *Candida* infection, 139
Testicular appendage, torsion of, 121
Testicular torsion, 107, 120–121
Tetanus vaccine, 158, 159, 162, 169
Thompson test, 160
Thoracentesis, 46–47
Thrombocytopenic purpura, 30–31
Thrombolytics, in pulmonary embolism, 55
Thrombosis, venous, 24–25
Thrombotic thrombocytopenic purpura, 30–31
Thyroid-stimulating hormone, in palpitations, 18
Tinel's sign, 172
Toothache, 100–101
Torsion
 ovarian, 126–127
 testicular, 107, 120–121
 testicular appendage, 121
Transesophageal echocardiography, in aortic dissection, 3
Trichomoniasis, 138
Tuberculosis, 48

U

Ulcer, peptic, 74, 82–83
Ultrasonography
 in abdominal aortic aneurysm, 58
 in abdominal pain, 189
 in acute renal failure, 105
 in appendicitis, 61
 in biliary disease, 64
 in ectopic pregnancy, 124–125
 in ovarian torsion, 126
 in pulmonary embolism, 55
 of scrotum, 110, 121
 in spontaneous abortion, 134
 in vaginal bleeding, 137
 in venous thrombosis, 24
Umbilical hernia, 109
Unstable angina, 22–23
Urethritis, gonococcal, 119

Urinalysis, 114, 117
Urinary tract infection, 114–115
Urine, alkalinization of, 117
Urticaria, 184–185

V

Vaccine
 Hemophilus influenza, 98
 rabies, 159
 tetanus, 158, 159, 162, 169
Vaginal bleeding, 136–137
Vaginosis, 138, 139
Varicocele, 110–111
Vasculitis, urticarial, 185
Vasopressin, in gastrointestinal bleeding, 75
Vena cava filter, 55
Venous thrombosis, 24–25
Ventilation/perfusion scan, in pulmonary embolism, 55
Ventricular fibrillation, 6–7
Ventricular tachycardia, 6–7, 19
Vertigo, 152–153
Viral infection. *See* Infection
Virchow's triad, 55
Vomiting, pregnancy-related, 128
Vulvovaginitis, 138–139

W

Warts, genital, 119
Weakness, 154–155
Wernicke's encephalopathy, 39
Westermark sign, 54
Whipple's triad, 39
Wrist pain, 172–173

X

X-ray
 in abdominal aortic aneurysm, 59
 in ankle sprain, 160
 in bowel obstruction, 62–63
 in diverticulitis, 68
 of fracture, 164
 in ischemic bowel, 78
 in laceration, 168
 in low back pain, 171
 in rhabdomyolysis, 117
 of teeth, 101
X-rays
 in abdominal pain, 189
 chest. *See* Chest x-ray

Y

Yeast infection, 138, 139

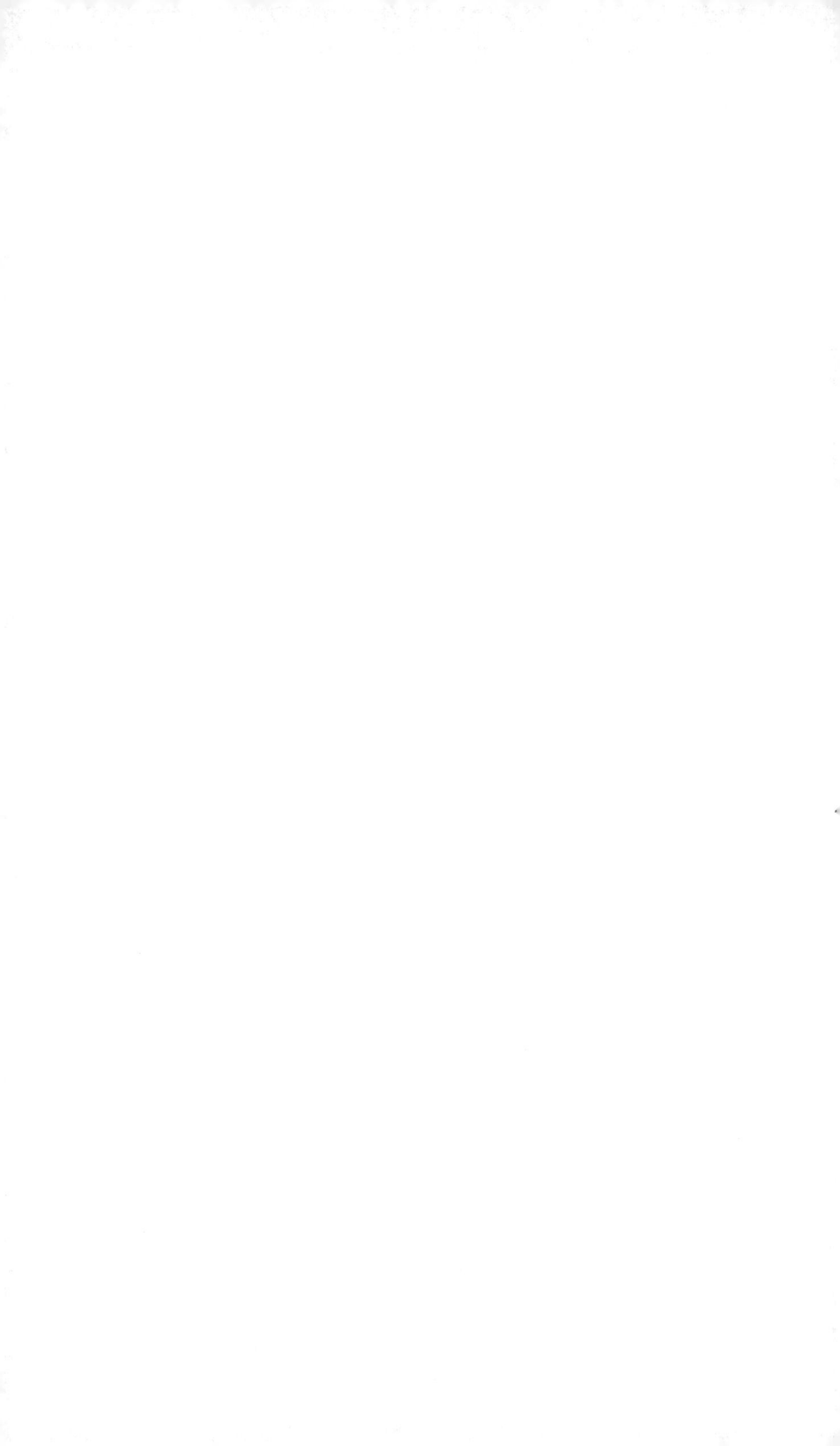